MORE PRAISE FOR

Julie Motz

"With warmth, humor and well-paced prose, she offers a fascinating look at her work, her patients and the ways her techniques can be adapted for everyday self-discoveries."
—*Publishers Weekly*

"Julie Motz has captured the essence of mind-body medicine at the cellular level. This is a must read for any open-minded person suffering from an illness."
—Stephen Sinatra, M.D., author of *Optimum Health*

"Extraordinary stories of her experience helping patients to handle their surgeries and to heal themselves afterward."
—*Common Boundary*

"Julie Motz provides a fascinating look at her unique, powerful synergy of medicine and healing."
—Mitch Gaynor, M.D., Director, Strang Cancer Prevention Center

"More than anything else, what Motz offers critically ill patients is a human touch."
—*Country Living's Healthy Living*

Utne Reader cited Julie Motz's hands-on healing work as one of "15 ideas that could shake the world" (March/April 1999 issue).

BANTAM
BOOKS

New York Toronto London
Sydney Auckland

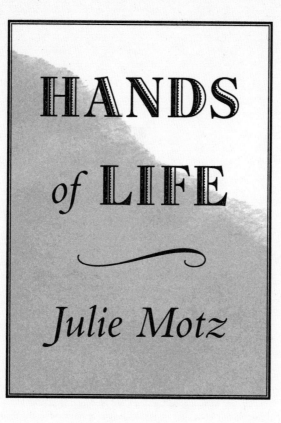

HANDS of LIFE

Julie Motz

Use Your Body's
Own Energy Medicine for
Healing, Recovery, and
Transformation

This edition contains the complete text
of the original hardcover edition.
NOT ONE WORD HAS BEEN OMITTED.

HANDS OF LIFE
A Bantam Book

PUBLISHING HISTORY
Bantam hardcover edition published September 1998
Bantam trade paperback edition / March 2000

Book design by Laurie Jewell.

ISBN: 0-553-37925-9

Published simultaneously in the United States and Canada

Bantam Books are published by Bantam Books, a division of Random
House, Inc. Its trademark, consisting of the words "Bantam Books" and the
portrayal of a rooster, is Registered in U.S. Patent and Trademark Office
and in other countries. Marca Registrada. Bantam Books, 1540 Broadway,
New York, New York 10036.

PRINTED IN THE UNITED STATES OF AMERICA
BVG   10   9   8   7   6   5   4   3   2   1

CONTENTS

*This book is dedicated to
Patrick Gilligan, in loving memory,
and to my parents,
Lloyd and Minne Motz.*

ACKNOWLEDGMENTS

I would like to thank the very bright and insightful editor of this book, Brian Tart; my extraordinary agent, Janis Vallely; and my thoughtful and caring editor at *Advances,* Harris Dienstfrey. I would also like to thank Sonja Gilligan for all her love and encouragement and my wonderful friend Michelle Clifton, who has been asking me for years, "When are you going to write the book, Julie?"

Chapter One

INTO THE
OPERATING ROOM

It has been eight months since I first walked through the doors of the department of cardiothoracic surgery of Columbia Presbyterian Medical Center in upper Manhattan. The department has its suite of elegant offices in one wing of the seventh floor of the center's newest building, and patients recovering from its highly technical and remunerative surgeries occupy another. It has been five months since I began treating some of these patients, using the energy that flows through my hands to help them heal the terrible and awesome things that have happened inside their chests. It has been a month since I first met George, the patient who will change my life.

For a while, just to be doing such healing work, and to have it be effective in the highly mechanized and computerized realm of academic medicine, where machines extend life beyond anybody's wildest dreams, was mystery and challenge enough. But for the past few weeks I have been in the grip of an obsession about the operating room. If I can be effective after surgery, what might I accomplish if I could run energy into these open and wounded bodies while the transformation under the surgeon's knife is actually occurring?

I don't bother to think about the fact that this has never been done before—the idea seems to me so natural, such an obvious extension of what I am already doing. I don't bother to think that what I'm doing already seems odd enough to the nurses and the attending cardiologists on the unit—and even to Dr. Mehmet Oz, the surgeon whose patients I am treating.

What I think about are scalpels and saws cutting through unresisting flesh and bone, and pieces of anatomy being removed and rearranged, and the surrender to this invasion that the patient must endure. And I think about the energy in the room—the collective passions of surgeon and patient, each needing this process to succeed, but for different reasons.

The more I think about it, the more I am convinced that I belong there.

In part, I am fueled by my own habitual reaction to resistance—which is, when something is denied me, to press even harder for something even more difficult and out of reach. My first mild suggestion to Dr. Oz that I follow him into the OR "just to see what the energy is like" met with an easy "Sure, any time." This was followed a week later by a declaration that something like a dispensation from the pope would probably be required.

"Why the change?" I ask myself. And then I think of what I know about Dr. Oz—a young ambitious man on an incredibly fast track, with a glut of papers already published and more on the way. Something in the prevailing political winds must have wafted by and told him that this was not the time to be seen bringing an utterly civilian "New Age" healer into the operating room. The moment he had a change of heart, however, something in me ratcheted up the stakes. It would not be enough just to be there as an observer. I would have to work on a patient while he was undergoing surgery.

And now, because of George, I just might have a chance. A

handsome, virile Vietnam navy veteran, he is a favorite of Dr. Oz's because his case is so difficult; death had seemed almost certain when they first met in the cardiac critical care unit. "He wasn't going to operate," George told me. "I was that sick. But I said, 'Hey, I've been to Vietnam, and I know I'm not going to die on any operating table. Go ahead.'"

And so Dr. Oz performed the very tricky, very dangerous surgery. He put into George's body a huge hunk of metal, operated by an outside pump, that took over the work of the left ventricle of his heart, called an LVAD (for "left ventricle assist device").

My own relationship with George began after that surgery, in the cardiac intensive care unit—a kind of minipurgatory between surgery and recovery or death. In its dim light, nurses watch their immobile patients through glass doors and keep the television sets in the patient cubicles running all the time, often muttering over the objections of the inert forms in the beds, "It's good for you—they've done a study." I am struck by the fact that George has succeeded in getting someone to turn his TV off.

I am also struck by his pale good looks, his utter weariness, and his wry skepticism. Even more impressive is his ability to give himself over to the work we do together. "I didn't believe in any of this stuff when I first met you, Julie," he says. "But when the surgeon who has saved your life suggests something, you give it a try."

"Would you be willing to try me in the operating room, George?" I ask. Of course he would.

A week after that conversation, I find Dr. Oz eating lunch in his office. He offers me some and, when I decline, pushes a bag of luminously orange dried apricots across the desk in my direction. "From Turkey," he says. "A friend of my father's keeps sending them. So what's new?"

"I'd like to be there, in the operating room, when you do George's transplant," I say, and hold my breath. I can see the computer circuits clicking inside his brain, spitting out the answer to him in seconds. "Hm," he frowns, stops chewing and pretends to give it some thought, while his dark eyes go totally blank. Then, "Yeah, yeah—why not?" Amazed and relieved, I run to tell George the good news. He smiles at me knowingly, as if to say, "I told you it would be okay." It makes me wonder if he has already asked Dr. Oz himself.

Walking back from George's room, I begin to contemplate what the response of the other people in the OR might be to the sight of a strange masked woman standing with her hands on the patient's head and whispering into his supposedly unhearing ears. It occurs to me (knowing nothing about cardiac surgery, and assuming, quite mistakenly, that the same people work there all the time) that it might be a good idea for me to introduce myself to them beforehand and thereby reduce the potential for shock.

Accordingly, I ask Dr. Oz and he agrees. Since George's surgery will occur as soon as a suitable heart shows up, and that heart could be as near as the next traffic accident on the West Side Highway (which George can see from his room), there is no time to lose. Dr. Oz has a coronary bypass scheduled for that afternoon, and we go down the escalators to the operating-room suite together. He punches in the code that allows the door to the surgical inner sanctum to open.

He leads me to the racks where blue scrub suits, masks, shower caps, and shoe coverings are stacked, then disappears behind a door through which I can hear men's voices and then laughter, as if someone has just told a joke. I enter the one marked "Women's Dressing Room," with the paraphernalia of his profession he has handed me clutched against my chest.

The dressing room where the OR nurses and the few women surgeons change is filled with rows of banged-up lockers. Discarded scrubs and masks lie on wooden benches. Dr. Oz has told me that he doesn't wear any underwear under his scrub suit "because it just gets covered with blood." I decide to keep mine on, however, and pull the drawstring pants and the shirt on over it. I meet him again in the corridor between the two dressing rooms. He shows me how to pinch the top of my mask so it stays up on my nose, and I follow him through a series of passageways and a set of swinging doors into the cube of unnaturally bright and beeping space that is the operating room.

It is freezing—cold enough to make me wish I had two sets of underwear, or two sets of scrubs on. I wonder if this would seem "unprofessional" or simply unmacho. I wonder if, in this arena, the two are the same.

To my surprise, the surgery seems already well under way. I later learn that Dr. Oz often does not "open" for himself, unless it is one of the trickier cases, like a mechanical heart implant, or a transplant involving a patient already on a mechanical heart. The preliminary work—in this case, painting the body with betadine, a disinfectant the color of dried blood, draping the sterile blue cloths around the area of the incision, cutting into the chest and sawing open the sternum, and even opening the leg to remove the veins that will take over the work of the coronary arteries—has already been done by a surgical resident.

I expect to just take a quick look around, introduce myself, and then leave, but Dr. Oz motions me to go stand at the head of the patient, as he disappears through a set of swinging doors opposite the ones through which we have entered. Stepping in front of the anesthesiologist, I realize that I am expected to watch the surgery—something I hadn't quite counted on.

In two minutes Dr. Oz is back, his hands dripping. A contraption like a miniature miner's lamp, with high-powered binocular spectacles attached, is strapped to his head. He dives into the surgical gloves the nurse holds out for him, and slips into the sterile gown, which she ties behind him. He positions himself on the right side of the body, with his back to a machine that powers the lamp's high-intensity beam.

Virtually nothing of the patient is visible except the gaping wetness of her chest. I deduce that there is a woman under all the draping from the wisps of hair that I can just barely see protruding from the sides of her cap. I take a deep breath and look into the blood-filled space. I have never witnessed a surgery before, but I feel fortified by having seen a video that Dr. Oz lent me a few weeks before, of a mechanical heart implant procedure. I was able to watch the whole thing without turning my head away once. Very promising for someone who could never stand the sight of blood, I thought.

While Dr. Oz uses a tiny electric torch to cut closer to the heart, I notice the resident holding something in the air that looks like a worm but that I know must be a vein. And then it happens—I hear, with what set of ears I do not know, the vein screaming in terror. The brain, shut down and furious, begins muttering "nobody told me about this, nobody told me about this, nobody told me about this," like a mantra. The heart, without blood or pulse, is moaning in confusion and pain.

I look around me. I check out the surgical nurse, passing instruments to the surgeons; the circulating nurse, moving between the sterile and nonsterile fields; the perfusionists, monitoring the heart-lung machine; the attending and resident anesthesiologists, busy writing notes; Dr. Oz and the surgical resident, peering into and poking away at the chest cavity. Nobody seems to notice a thing. Everybody is proceeding briskly, if not exactly cheerfully, with his or her task, as if this emotional cacophony were not going on.

I wonder if I'm going crazy—and then I think about all the messages I have received from people's bodies over the years in which I have worked as an energy healer. I know that this ability to tune in and hear or feel what is going on inside them is one of the reasons people come to me for healing. But this is different. I have never heard a part of a body screaming, muttering, or moaning before.

What strikes me at the moment is how totally unprepared the body seems to be for what is happening to it. No one has warned the vein that it is going to be removed from its cozy, familiar position in the leg, with sluggish venous blood oozing comfortably through it, to take up duty as a coronary artery, sustaining the fast, throbbing flow of arterial blood. No one has told the brain that muscles will not respond to the frantic messages it sends firing down the nerves, or that it will have to nourish itself for an hour or more on chilled blood treated with a special chemical to keep it from clotting in the machine. No one has told the heart that it must lie quietly for a while, during which time its whole reason for being, the movement of blood through the body, will be taken over by an external device. And no one has thanked the body, either in parts or as a whole, for its courage in undergoing this ordeal.

Realizing that this is not a suitable time to bring these subjects up for discussion—realizing, in fact, that there may never be a suitable time to talk to anyone at the hospital about any of this—I refocus my attention on the mechanical details of the surgery. I stare with fascination at the blood coming out of the patient's body through heavy tubing and swirling through the heart-lung machine, which cleanses it of waste and reoxygenates it before it journeys back again. Immediately I think of the possibilities of training the people who run the machine to treat the blood energetically as it goes through. ("It wouldn't work," Dr. Oz tells me later. "They're just blue-collar workers. They wouldn't even understand what you're talking about. In fact, they'd probably laugh at you.") I continue to marvel at my own ability to watch all this without flinching. But just as I am congratulating myself, just as I hear Dr. Oz, who is now delicately sewing the vein into place on the heart, say, "I don't know what I would have done if they hadn't invented vicryl stitches," every cell in my body seems to go into revolt. I feel as if I've just taken my fifth drink (about two past my limit), and a strange, spiral motion travels through my limbs, loosening my brain's control over them. Or perhaps my brain has finally put two and two together and realized what it is recording—the bloody inner workings of a sawed-open human being, not too terribly different, anatomically, from myself.

"Mehmet," I say, just loudly enough to get his attention, "I have to go now."

"Are you okay?" he asks, a little surprised.

"Quite frankly, no." I manage to mutter, between clenched teeth.

"Get her a chair, get her a chair!" he yells.

"No," I say, knowing that to exit the scene entirely is my only salvation. "I have to leave the room."

I feel the comforting grasp of someone at my elbow, and a burly perfusionist gently ushers me out into the corridor, somehow managing to support the weight that my legs can't quite seem to balance on top of them. I don't know exactly where he's leading me, but suddenly we are standing in front of a gurney, and I manage to lift myself up onto it and collapse.

The cells in my body continue to spin and spin, as I stare at the ceiling in despair. Any hopes I had of a life as a healer in the operating room have suddenly evaporated. I would hardly be of much help to the patients, slumped in a heap on the floor.

Just as I am thinking my glummest thoughts, a cheerful spirit appears at my side. It is the other perfusionist, Jery Whitworth, a former nurse with a long-standing interest in alternative therapies. "How are you doing?" he asks.

"Just awful," I moan. "What am I going to do about this?"

"Not to worry," he says, confidently. "The first time I watched open heart, I collapsed onto a rolling stool and went zooming across the operating room floor. It happens to a lot of us. You'll be fine."

"But how?"

"Easy. I'll desensitize you."

"Oh, great, thanks," I say, not knowing what in the world he has in mind.

In about an hour I find I can stagger to my feet without the distressing sense that every part of me wants to travel in a different direction. Luckily I have no more patients scheduled for treatment that day, so I drive home, which takes about an hour.

Exhausted, I go to bed early, with visions of Jery leading me closer and closer to an operating table over which Dr. Oz stands with scalpel, torch, or saw held ready and waiting. *Desensitize,* I think, savoring the word, as I drift off the sleep.

I awaken with a jolt to the ringing of the telephone. It is the LVAD coordinator. "We have a heart for George. He goes down at one."

I look at the clock. It is eleven-thirty. I will have just enough time, perhaps without even speeding, to make it.

My own heart is pounding fast enough to make me a candidate for one of Dr. Oz's procedures. I drive down the almost empty highway, too excited to listen to the radio or tapes. I keep seeing George, with those thick tubes coming out of his side, and the machine they are connected to, pumping life through his body.

As I turn off the highway, my stomach suddenly comes up into my throat. *My God!* I think. *How the hell am I going to keep from fainting?*

A coward's voice whispers into my ear to just turn around and go home. I could say I got a flat tire. I could say the car wouldn't start. I could say anything, anything at all, to spare myself the humiliation of ending up in a collapsed heap underneath the operating table. But I have promised George that I will be there. It is only as I am walking up the hill from Riverside Drive to the hospital, its huge buildings looming above the tenements that surround it, that I devise a plan. Since my work during the surgery will involve channeling energy through my hands into the patient's body, there is no reason that I actually have to watch anything that is going on. Once I've positioned myself at his head, with my hands on either side, I can just stare at the ceiling. Hopefully everybody else in the room will be so preoccupied with their immediate tasks that no one will notice the oddness of this posture.

Enormously relieved and pleased with myself, I do not even worry about what eight hours of this neck-craning activity might do to the equanimity of my upper spine. I flash my pass at the security guard and take the elevator to the seventh floor, just in time to find George as he is being moved from his bed to a gurney. I give him a hug and feel fear alternating with excitement in his chest.

When I see him again about ten minutes later, I am masked and in scrubs in the operating room, and he is being wheeled through its doors, into the intensely illuminated coldness where the miracle designed to save his life is being prepared. By this time, fear has taken over. I feel it coming in great waves off his body, although he keeps smiling and telling everyone how calm he is. I marvel, as I will often do again, at the patient's need to take care of the feelings of his doctors.

Without contradicting George's protestations of calmness, and hopefully without embarrassing him, I abandon all my fancy plans for working on various acupuncture points on his feet to stimulate certain organs, and I simply hold his hand as the needles for the intravenous lines go in. He is sweating, in spite of the coldness of the room, and as I look into his eyes, I try to let the tension of his body ease itself through mine. The anesthesiologist is brisk and competent but not particularly interested in a feeling connection with the patient. "Task oriented" is the best phrase to describe the attitude of a typical surgical team.

The insertion of the needles into the arm is only mildly painful, but inserting the Swan-Gantz catheter is agony. This is a tube, inserted without anesthesia, into the pulmonary artery, through the right side of the neck. George's face is covered as the incision is made, which seems to increase his anxiety. The catheter is pushed through the blood vessel, down into the heart, where it will stay throughout the entire surgery, measuring the pressure from the two left chambers. As the flat lines in a screen behind begin to wave and spike, the Swan is taped into place and a mask is brought down over George's face.

"This is just oxygen," the anesthesiologist tells him. "Breathe deeply, and in a little while you'll be drifting off to sleep." This is not true, of course. As the EEG will record, the brain waves of someone under anesthesia are very different from those of someone who is asleep. And as I will discover, this is not a time of peaceful dreams.

When George finally succumbs, jelly is put on his eyelids, and his eyes are taped closed to keep them from being damaged and from drying out during the surgery. A breathing tube is pushed down his trachea and taped in place around his mouth. Then an ultrasound camera is pushed down the esophagus. Once it is in position, black-and-white images of some pulsing shape I am told is his heart appear on the screen.

The anesthesiologist assures the surgical fellow who will be assisting Dr. Oz that George is immobile and, for their purposes, "unconscious." The sheet and gown that have covered him are removed, and I am struck by the vulnerability and beauty of his inert body. Icy cold pads that are used to ground the Bovies—the electric torches that do most of the work once done by scalpels—are slapped on his sides, and a catheter is inserted into his penis, as is common in most long surgeries. Its output will be a measure of how well the kidneys, which are in critical partnership with the heart, are doing.

All sense of this being a "person" seems to have vanished from the room, and I am struck by the thought that we turn the body into a machine in order to work on it with machines. Betadine is applied by the surgical fellow, just as Dr. Oz steps into the room, hands dripping from the scrub sink.

Once dried, gowned, and gloved, he proceeds to the side of the operating table, and I notice that some distinct change has occurred in the energy in the room. Some sense of purpose and profound caring has suddenly suffused the atmosphere, and I am struck by the tenderness (there is no other word for it) with which he lays the sterile blue cloths all around the area on which he will operate.

The scrub nurse hands him the scalpel, and I look away, just as the first trickle of blood oozes onto George's groin. The bypass may have to be done through the femoral artery and vein, instead of in the usual fashion, through the aorta and the right atrium. Standing with my hands on George's temples, I am surprised that his energy feels just as vital to me as on the previous occasions when we have worked together. Under general anesthesia, unless an effort is made to ground the energy field—that is to say, draw it down toward the feet—the energy tends to concentrate itself around the head. This is a phenomenon as mysterious and unexplained in the world of energy medicine as the mechanisms of anesthesia itself are in the more conventional world of chemical medicine.

Staring at the ceiling, I hear the buzz of the Bovie, which cuts through flesh and, in a perfect surgical world, seals off blood vessels as it does so. After a few hours, the sizzling fat and muscle will perfume the air with the incongruous scent of an outdoor barbecue, but for now there is just the *zzzzzz*, as Dr. Oz dissects the artery and the vein free of surrounding tissue. I also feel a strange kind of cringing in my own genital area, as if I were withdrawing from some kind of wound there. I later learn that George's plans for having children with his current wife, Susan, were cruelly aborted by the onset of his heart condition, and that their great hope is that the transplant will put their plans for creating a family back on track.

As Dr. Oz moves up the table to open the chest, I look down at George's body again and keep my eyes there until Dr. Oz reaches for the electric saw. Staring at the ceiling, I hear it whine its way through the wires that have held George's sternum together since the last surgery. Then there is the *plink, plink* of the wires being removed and dropped into a steel basin. Curiosity overcomes instincts of self-preservation, and I find my-self staring down into the cavity of his chest, held open by two steel clamps that have been inserted on either side of the ster-num and ratcheted back with a hand crank.

For the next nine hours (the surgery turns out to be longer than expected), this is where my attention remains focused, with no hint of the faintness and dizziness I had been dreading. Somehow my brain, given permission not to look, has adjusted to the extraordinary sight before it: a chest with its protective armor sawed in two, its precious contents exposed to the air, and human hands moving around inside it, cutting and burning to reach their goal, destroying in order to heal.

Inside the cavity Dr. Oz continues to work with the Bovie. Although all I can see of his face are his eyes, and they are fo-cused away from me on the bloody tissue he is probing with his hands, I can feel a sense of growing frustration rising inside him. "Can't find tissue plane," he says, apparently to no one in par-ticular.

"What?" I ask, uncertain of both what I have heard and what it could mean.

"I can't find the damn heart!" he says. Then he explains that the body has created an enormous amount of scar tissue in and around the LVAD, making it very difficult to find the border of the heart. Finally, he decides to go in through the peritoneal cavity, near the stomach, reaching up under George's diaphragm with his fingers.

A call is put through to the OR from the surgeons at the hospital where the donor heart is still in its nineteen-year-old body. They want to know if Dr. Oz is ready yet to have it "har-vested." The timing couldn't be worse, since over an hour has been lost with Oz searching for the tissue plane, and he is con-scious of the lag. "Tell them no—not yet. We'll call them." He knows very well that the longer the heart spends outside its fa-miliar surroundings of flesh and blood, the less vitality it will have when it reaches the patient. He also knows that the surgeons poised and waiting by the body of the donor are tired and would like to get the job over with and go home.

This is not likely to happen soon, because the adhesions are making it difficult for him to separate the heart from the pericardium, the sac of connective tissue that surrounds it and helps protect it from shock. While he is struggling to do this, another call comes from the donor end, and he says in frustration, "Not until I tell them!"

I have not taken my eyes from the opening in George's chest, but from the moment Dr. Oz's gloved fingers actually touched his heart, I have been experiencing something peculiar in my own. First there is a sense of churning anger and pain, and then the feeling of something struggling to break free. Suddenly an image comes to me of a much younger George, fending off blows from other boys. There is a very clear feeling of having to be tough and not show any pain. And also a feeling of humiliation and defeat, as if defending himself were of no use. When I mention this to him after the surgery, he immediately relates it to his experiences playing football.

I lean over and whisper in his ear that anger is an appropriate feeling to be having, and that he needs it to get through the challenges of the surgery. I also tell him that this time he will not be beaten down but that he will win. The sensation in my chest subsides, the image fades, and a calm determination seems to take over his motionless form.

At last enough of the heart is dissected free for Dr. Oz to allow the donor heart to be explanted and for George to be put "on bypass." That is to say, through the tubes inserted in the femoral artery and vein, blood will now bypass his heart and lungs, flowing through a machine that removes waste gases, like carbon dioxide, and puts oxygen back in. It is this miraculous piece of technology that allows most open heart surgery to be done without killing the patient.

It does, however, have a down side. For reasons no one understands, blood seems to get sticky from traveling through the machine, and so a chemical called heparin is added to it to allow it to move smoothly when it is returned to the body. Perhaps because the brain doesn't like this particular chemical, or perhaps because it just senses something disquietingly unfamiliar about the blood from its extracorporeal journeying, there is a high risk of postoperative depression, usually correlated with time spent "on the pump." This and other disruptions to the system that are better observed than explained, make one of the goals of the surgery to minimize the amount of time the patient must depend on the bypass machine for the flow of life.

Since the machine is now taking over for both the heart and the lungs, the LVAD can safely be disconnected. It is no longer needed to do the work of George's diseased left ventricle. Dr. Oz then uses the Bovie to clear the remaining adhesions between the heart and the chest wall, explaining to me that it was his anticipation of this complication that made him choose the blood vessels in the groin for the entry and exit points of blood going to the machine, rather than the usual choices of aorta and right atrium of the heart.

As he is clearing the adhesions, something that looks like an oversize Styrofoam picnic hamper is brought into the room. I glance at it longingly, realizing that it contains George's new heart. I would love to go over and put my hands on it, to feel the energy of the new organ and to send supporting energy into it. But I don't dare. I'm afraid it would look just a little too odd and make people too uncomfortable.

Dr. Oz continues to work at freeing the heart, and a sense of sadness comes into my chest when he has succeeded. I cannot tell if the sorrow is George's, the heart's, or both. The LVAD is then removed from the body, and I watch as the piece of hollow metal that has lived inside George and given him life for almost two months is handed off the sterile field of the surgery. Although each of these devices costs $40,000 to produce, they are never reused. Instead, each one is taken apart and studied.

Tissue that has adhered to or grown inside it is cultured and analyzed. While the device has been approved by the FDA for use in certain restricted situations (only if mortality is imminent within forty-eight hours and no transplant organ is available), it is still considered highly experimental.

Dr. Oz is now handed George's new heart, with a piece of the aorta attached. He makes a few incisions in the aorta to widen it and allow a better fit with George's primary artery. It, too, seems full of sorrow, although without being able to put my hands near it, I can't determine the cause. He then carefully stitches the heart in place and next instructs the perfusionist (the technician operating the bypass machine) to allow warmed blood to come into George's new heart. Tiny pricks are made in the heart to release air pockets before George comes fully "off bypass."

George's head starts to feel warmer to my touch, and I realize that it has been quite cold for some time. In the excitement of trying to absorb everything going on around me, I hadn't noticed the temperature drop when the bypass circulation was started. I later learn that while the patient is on the pump, the blood temperature is brought down to retard the body's metabolism and brain function. It is thought that this slowing of the body's clock makes the procedure less disruptive.

With the new heart in place and beating and George safely off the bypass machine, there is a noticeable drop in the tension in the room. The focus is now on preventing internal hemorrhaging, and Dr. Oz and the surgical fellow assisting him work with Bovies to cauterize any "bleeders." The chest cavity is repeatedly washed out with saline solution, and finally all seems to be well. The ratchet that has held George's sternum and rib cage open is released, the clamps are removed, and steel wires with curved needles at either end, sharp and strong enough to pierce bone, are passed through either side of his sternum. When all of these are in place, the ends of each are twisted together, clipped, and bent over, as close to the bone as possible. Watching Dr. Oz draw George's chest together like this, I am struck by the utter, almost crude physicality of surgical procedures.

I watch the surgical fellow stitching flesh to flesh and then skin to skin together, after Dr. Oz has left and thanked us all. There is a decided letdown in the room. George's incision is dressed, someone calls for a gurney, and he is transferred from the operating table to the stretcher. Knowing that he will not be conscious for at least twelve hours, I do not follow him into the ICU. Once he is gone, I notice with some surprise what a very ordinary room we have been working in—just a brightly lit box with two sets of swinging doors and some equipment. All its specialness seems gone. It is not even like a stage after the actors have departed and the scenery is struck, because that setting always seems to imply some kind of impending drama, and this does not.

It's as if the very space in the room were some kind of vacuum, sucking up all remnants of human feeling, like the suctioning tubes Dr. Oz uses to draw blood out of the area in which he is working. It seems a room without ghosts or memories, although many, many dramas, both triumphant and fatal, have been played out here.

I drive home, up along the Hudson River, in broad daylight, thinking about George and hoping for the best for him. A few days later I go to see him in the cardiac surgical ICU, where we first met. He has been having trouble making urine, and I put my thumbs on an acupuncture point at the bottom of each foot that the Chinese call Bubbling Spring. It is the starting point of the kidney meridian and is just at the center of the bottom of the ball of the foot. In Chinese medical theory it is believed that every time we walk, we take energy in from the earth through this point. From here it travels up to the kidneys, which they often visualize as two little feet at the back of our bodies, under the rib cage, pushing us along through life.

The functional description of the kidneys in Chinese medicine seems to include the adrenal glands as well, which sit right above them. The kidneys are considered key organs for supplying and balancing the body's energy, but they have another purpose as well. There is, in classical Chinese medicine, no psychology apart from physiology. That is to say, all emotions are believed to be carried in the energy of specific organs, and the brain, as an organ, is not even discussed. It is simply an outgrowth (or an ingrowth, if you will) of the skull.

The primary emotion of the kidneys is fear. But they are also believed to be the seat of deep sorrow. So someone suffering from either unabatable terror or profound emotional pain might be treated with herbs that were tonic to the kidneys, or with needles placed at various points on the kidney meridian. Physical damage to the kidneys might inhibit someone's ability to endure fear or sorrow, or the intense suppression of either feeling might damage these organs.

I think about this as I work on George simply by touching those points and bringing my awareness there. This alone seems to allow energy, which we both feel, to pass through me, from some as yet undiscovered source. Years of experience have taught me that I am certainly not the source, because I am never tired or depleted after working. On the contrary, I almost always feel energized myself. I believe that when you touch someone with a loving or healing intention, you create a kind of energy magnet that draws energy to the place you were touching. Similarly, when you think about someone or a part of his body, the energy of your thought draws ambient energy there.

First I suggest that he send the energy his kidneys were absorbing into his bladder. Ever since George and I healed a bedsore of his together by sending the blocked energy in the area down his leg, he has been both adept and enthusiastic at moving energy in his body. Then I remember the sorrow I experienced from his new heart in the operating room. I suggest that he honor this by connecting that sorrow with his kidneys and then allowing it to flow with the energy from the kidneys into the bladder and out from his body.

When I return a week later, George is back up on the seventh floor. He tells me that his kidney function and urine production normalized the day I saw him, and that his first biopsy revealed that he was not rejecting his new heart. He also tells me that his heart rate was almost normal after the surgery—a very unusual occurrence. The bad news is that his blood pressure has been dropping precipitously, and no one can figure out why.

I put my hands lightly on the tops of his feet, with nothing particular in mind, and immediately get the image of a small boy with his arm around a dog. "Did you have a pet when you were a kid?" I ask him.

"Yes," he says.

"What was it?"

"A dog." I can feel, with this response, a slight tightening in his throat.

"What happened to it?" I ask.

"My parents gave it away—without asking me."

"What was its name?"

"King," he says.

"I see." My hands, still resting on his feet, are starting to tingle. "I'm going to make a suggestion to you, George. I want you to take a deep breath, and as you exhale, I want you to say in a high, little boy's voice, 'Good-bye, King.' "

He takes a deep breath. "Good-bye, King," he says, almost singing the words.

"Again," I say.

"Good-bye, King." Tears are now running down his cheeks, and my shoulders suddenly let go and relax. I have him repeat this a few more times, and we both start to vibrate internally with the energy of his sorrow.

I realize that George has been trying to "protect" his new heart from his sadness, and that his life's training has been to take care of other people's pain but never his own. "You can't withhold your pain from your new heart, George," I tell him. "It needs to know everything about you, including how you've been hurt."

When I visit him a week later, he smiles proudly at me as I walk into the room. "It worked," he says. "My blood pressure stabilized twenty minutes after you left. And do you know what I did that night? I stayed up and told the whole story of my life to my heart."

That day each of the four other LVAD patients I work with asks me shyly if I will "do for them what I did for George." I am moved and flattered by their trust and their hope. My hope is that they can somehow befriend their own bodies, as George has done, and that each will enter into the mysteries of the flesh with enthusiasm and curiosity instead of terror and despair.

Chapter Two

DISCOVERING
HANDS OF LIFE

My own journey into energy healing has been an attempt over decades to truly inhabit my body, although this was not at all clear to me when that journey began. It started one February night in 1970 with my introduction to Fusion Groups, in the heyday of the human potential movement. The current glut of tabloid talk shows, in which everything is being shoved out of the closet and into our faces is, I believe, the cultural residue of this movement, and basically a healthy one. But before Oprah there was Synanon and its many offspring; and before nationally syndicated show-and-tell, there was the encounter group.

Run by Mike and Sonja Gilligan, Fusion Groups were a brilliant and effective example of this genre; the basic format involved fifteen to twenty-five people, including the two group leaders, sitting in a circle. After going around once with names, someone would "ask for the involvement" of the group and talk about some aspect of his life for which he wanted support or help. The person speaking would often not have a clear idea of what he was feeling about what he was saying, and it was the group's purpose, among other things, to supply this clarity.

I came into the groups at the suggestion of a fellow cinematography student at the graduate School of the Arts at Columbia University. I had missed ten days at the beginning of the semester because an episode with an overdose of sleeping pills had landed me in the emergency room, the ICU, and then the ward of the very hospital where I would later practice my healing skills. No one at school knew what had happened to me, but apparently the cloud of depression I walked around in when I came back was intense enough for someone who cared to notice.

My first direct experience of the group process (of which I was, for the first few weeks, a fascinated and terrified observer) came when someone in the group—a woman who was, not coincidentally, much like my mother—forgot my name when she was addressing me in the circle. I hadn't consciously allowed any feeling about this to register, when I suddenly heard Sonja's voice, very loud in my ear, although she was sitting halfway across the room: *"How do you feel when someone forgets your name, Julie?"* I stared at her blankly, my mouth dry, and couldn't think of anything to say. Except for an eerie sensation of being detached from everything in the room, including the chair I was sitting on, I wasn't aware of feeling anything. "I think you're angry," Sonja said, after what seemed like a gaping chasm of silence. "I have a knot in my stomach."

By a mechanism I did not yet understand but developed some theories about later, she was feeling in her own body my angry response to being slighted, which was, at the time, below the level of my own perception. Terror, almost tantamount to shock, was holding the anger at bay. Following Sonja's instructions, although I felt barely able to stand, I walked to a place in the circle facing a bare wall and visualized my mother standing in front of me. Taking a deep breath and making fists, I attempted to shout the word "Liar!" at her image. Twenty minutes later, after feeling I was going to faint or die, and after much encouragement from the group, I actually felt the strength of the anger moving through my body. I returned to my seat feeling more real than I had in months.

Six months before, I had finally gotten the courage to leave a man who was intensely jealous and physically abusive. I also left my old therapist, angry that she had not counseled me to get out of the affair. The new one to whom she referred me ended up seducing me, and the insanity of that affair had ended with the sleeping pills. During this period I had gone back to living with my parents and was thus thrust back into ancient terrors. I dealt with them by detaching myself emotionally through depression. On some profound level I was raging, as I had been for years, about the wounds inflicted on me as a child. Bulimia had been one method of deflecting this rage, but it hadn't been sufficient. When I wasn't depressed, I was paranoid, feeling that the world could fall in on me at any moment—that I had no substance, no reality. What I really was missing was a connection to the anger that could defend me and give me the energy to both ground myself and move forward.

That night in the group, for the first time I allowed my body to feel the power and the truth of my anger surging through me. I felt as I had not felt for many years—as if I belonged to the human race and to myself. My sense of being some kind of freak who couldn't feel or function the way other people could would not disappear completely for a long time. But I could smell freedom and sanity in the air—the freedom to feel, and the sanity of knowing exactly what I was feeling. It was intoxicating.

The Energy of Emotions

Anger was not the only feeling with which the encounter group concerned itself, although it appeared to be the one that most people had to experience fully in order to get to the other feelings. The Gilligans and others in the human potential movement were, I believe, the first people to identify anger as a good feeling—not something to be avoided, suppressed, or even gotten rid of but a necessary force of nature, to be felt, understood, and used.

Sonja Gilligan's unique contribution was to realize that there are four and only four basic feelings:

1. Fear is the same as excitement. It is the feeling state of perception. Fear tells you what is safe and what is dangerous, although we have been trained from childhood to identify it only with the perception of danger. Hate is the defensive form of fear.

2. Anger, negatively identified with a "kill" feeling, is the emotion of action. If your fear tells you that what you have perceived is safe, your anger carries you forward to get what you desire. If your fear tells you it is dangerous, your anger gives you the energy to fight or flee to protect yourself or what you value. Resentment is the defensive form of anger.

3. Pain, in the emotional sense, is self-knowledge. It is the feeling that comes up when you have either achieved what you have pursued or protected what you value and love. It puts you in touch with the core of your being and frequently moves you to tears (although people also cry to hide anger or fear). It also comes up when a loving feeling from someone else touches this core and reminds you where you live—a child's hug or a great artist's painting, poem, or symphony. Contempt is the defensive form of pain.

4. Love is the feeling that flows out from you, once you know who you are, to connect you to other people. It is sexuality and creativity. Joy is the defensive form of love.

The defensive form of a feeling is one that attaches itself to another feeling, so that we feel neither one clearly. We use the defensive form when the feeling itself seems too risky. After years of training ourselves to use defensive feelings, the defensive feelings often use us, taking over and denying us access to the basic feeling. Here is how it looks:

DEFENSIVE FORMS OF FEELING		
DEFENSIVE	COMBINATION OF FEELINGS	MESSAGE
Hate	= Fear + Anger	"Don't touch me."
Resentment	= Anger + Love	"You've hurt me."
Contempt	= Pain + Fear	"You can't hurt me because I'm above it all."
Joy	= Love + Pain	"You can't hurt me because nothing matters."

I was as fascinated with Sonja's theory as I was excited by the effects of the group process on my life. I became seized with a desire to understand how these forces called feelings manifest themselves on a physical level, and I made inquiries at the top biology research centers in the city: Rockefeller University, Columbia, and NYU. To my great disappointment, the physiology and biology of emotions wasn't on anybody's research agenda.

During this time I began to conclude that emotions are some kind of energy. After six months in those laboratories of emotions, the Fusion Groups, I found myself mysteriously endowed with the power to feel what other people were feeling, just as Sonja had done with me. Since I could do this over the telephone as well as face to face, visual clues did not seem to be a factor. Somehow feelings just traveled across space from someone else's body into mine. Even more interesting, this ability to feel other people's feelings—even feelings they didn't know they were having—was something that most people in the groups acquired in time. Apparently it was a skill that could be learned.

I believe that other people are giving us information about their emotions all the time (just as we are always in the process of having some emotion ourselves, even when we are sleeping). We're not trained to believe that these informational signals have any meaning or importance, so we usually don't focus on them. Occasionally when we are in the presence of someone with a great deal of unacknowledged or suppressed rage, we may feel extremely uncomfortable, or suddenly very sleepy, without knowing why. But the feelings are out there everywhere, all the time, available to everyone.

Learning to identify and interpret these physical signals as fear, anger, pain, or love is something like learning how to track with an Indian guide. At first, you are amazed that he can tell that a deer stood next to this particular tree, or that a fox came through the underbrush at just this point. Then the guide shows you the place where the buds have been stripped from a branch, or some dry leaves displaced along the path. It's not that you didn't "see" these things. They passed across your visual field, just as they did across his. But you didn't "notice" them, because you had not trained yourself to consider such signs as bearers of important information.

When I am teaching in a group, I will often stop and say something like "Can you feel what's going on in her back as she's talking?" This question brings the group's awareness to the place in that person's body where a blocked feeling is being held. The first time I ask, usually a couple of people nod. By the next session, about half are with me. By the third time we meet, usually everyone in the group of fifteen or twenty is picking it up. When people spend some time with me, they come into sync with me vibrationally and begin to use their bodies as emotional tuning forks the way I do, with greater and greater ease.

It was the French physicist Louis de Broglie who posited in the early part of this century that all matter emits waves, and that these matter waves (or de Broglie waves, as they came to be called) travel faster than the speed of light. To me it seems reasonable to assume that matter that is as highly organized as human tissue would not only give off distinctive and identifiable wave patterns but be able to receive and identify them. This is what I believe is going on when I feel another person's emotions in my body.

In the Gilligans' groups, feelings were dealt with on a whole-body level. Someone would say "You're angry" or "You're having a pain feeling." When Sonja would feel a knot in her stomach from someone else's unexpressed anger, or a dizziness in her head from their unrecognized fear, she didn't assume that they were actually experiencing the feeling in the same place—just that they were holding it in their body in some way. Fifteen years later, when I became a healer, I refined this work by taking it into the body in a much more specific way: relating it to disease and physical discomfort. I would get emotional messages from specific parts of the body, even parts of a cell, which were related to the ailment from which the patient was suffering.

When the Fusion Groups ended in 1971, I pursued my dream of being a filmmaker by forming a documentary film company with Mike and Sonja Gilligan and Chuck and Michelle Clifton, another couple from the groups. While feelings and energy were not the direct focus of my work, I had the benefit of being in daily contact with people who shared both the experience and the vocabulary that shaped my view of the mechanisms of human behavior.

How the Body Remembers

In 1982, in a freak accident, I fell and hurt my back in an acrobatics class, apparently injuring a few upper vertebrae in some vague undefined way. That is to say, after a lifetime of taking the perfect and effortless functioning of my body for granted, I became one of the vast number of Americans with intermittent back pain. My brother, a doctor, informed me that modern medicine could do nothing for me.

Not content to live with the pain, I followed the recommendations of friends with similar ailments and tales of miraculous cures. These led me first to an acupuncturist and then to a chiropractor, both of whom brought some but only temporary relief. I believe in the efficacy of their disciplines, but I also believe that in conventional and unconventional medicine alike, everything works for somebody and nothing works for everybody. I also believe that healing occurs at least as much through the relationship as through the technique, whatever the particular modality.

I had just about given up on finding a cure when I found myself at a dinner party in a fashionable section of Washington trying to describe my encounter group experiences. When I had finished, the host turned to his female companion, Janice, and said, "Have you ever told Julie about Reiki?" She hadn't.

What was it? I wanted to know. It turned out that Janice was in remission from ovarian cancer and attributed part of her recovery to a system of "energy healing" that had been brought here from Japan by way of Hawaii. Would it be effective for back pain? I wondered aloud, and the next thing I knew, I was being escorted from the dining room to the living room and instructed to lie facedown on the oriental carpet.

Janice knelt at my head and, in a quiet, very soothing voice, explained that she was going to place her hands at certain places on my back. Whenever she felt a coldness coming into one of her hands, which would indicate an energy deficiency, she would ask me to bring my awareness to that place in my body and to allow my mind to free-associate.

She then leaned over and put a hand on either shoulder blade. After about a minute, she said that she felt coldness in my left shoulder—which had, indeed, become quite stiff after the accident. Bring your awareness there, she instructed, and see what images come to mind. I had no idea what "bringing my awareness" to my shoulder meant, and so I just said to myself, *Be your shoulder, Julie.* In an instant I saw my mother, her face a contorted mask of rage, raising her hand to strike me across the face when I was six years old. I began to sob and shake. Then I heard Janice's voice saying, "I'm going to raise my hand from your shoulder, Julie, and pull the pain out." As she did so, the image faded and my crying stopped.

The rest of the treatment was soothing but uneventful, and I returned the next day to have Janice work on the front of my body. I left feeling deeply relaxed, as I had the night before. Riding home on the train, I had the distinct feeling that there was more space inside my shoulder than there had been before, as if the cells were taking deeper breaths and drawing more oxygen into the tissue. I had no way to explain any of what had happened to me, but that inability in no measure dampened my excitement about it.

Two things intrigued me about the memory that had so mysteriously and forcefully been thrust into my consciousness. The first was that I had always known that my mother used to hit me but had, until that time, no distinct image or sensory recall of any instances of her attacks, as if I had merely read some casual reference to them in a book. But last night I had reexperienced a specific attack, visually and viscerally, the feeling memory of which had been buried away.

The second was the connection of the memory to my shoulder. Only years later, talking about it to my niece, a physical therapist, did the pieces finally come together. "Your mother's right-handed, isn't she?" Nicole asked. "Then she would have hit you on the left side of your face. The natural impulse is to tighten your shoulder and bring it up to your chin to try to protect your face from the blow." I realized that my shoulder had also protected my brain from the full knowledge of what had happened to me by somehow holding that information for it. The shoulder knew in detail what the brain, in a moment of panic, had avoided knowing.

I have since witnessed this phenomenon in myself and in my patients, repeatedly, and over the years a few ideas about why it occurs have come to me. The most popular general theory about repression of emotionally charged memories is that the brain can't handle the information at the time the event occurs. Bonnie Bainbridge Cohen, founder of the School for Body-Mind Centering, believes that a protective mechanism keeps the neuronal circuits in the brain from being overloaded with traumatic information until the brain is ready to handle it. This mechanism stores the information in the motor neurons, which come off the front of the spinal cord, instead of allowing the impulses to travel up the neurons on the back of the spinal cord to the brain.

But why can't the brain be allowed to know that the body, or the spirit, has been hurt?

Before I encountered Bonnie's theory, I reasoned that the brain was making these decisions so that it could get on with its important job of running the world without having to stop for messy and time-consuming emotions. I sort of pictured it in the same relationship to the rest of the body as the human race is to all the other species on the planet. Nature gave it some tiny advantage, like a slightly greater blood flow, or a few more neurons, and now it thinks it's entitled to run the show. I pictured it as saying to a shoulder, or a knee, or a back, when some overwhelming wave of feeling started to come toward it, "You take it, Charlie, I'm too busy making this deal."

After many years of this treatment, of course, even faithful Charlie can't go on. "Listen," he says (usually in the form of weakness or pain), "I don't have enough energy to be a knee and hold this emotion for you at the same time. Since you're not willing to take the responsibility for registering this feeling, I'm going to have to give up being a knee."

I still think this is what happens, and I still think the purpose is protection, but for somewhat different reasons. The natural response to an injury is to be angry, and to take some action to defend oneself—like striking back, screaming for help, or running away. When a child who is injured by an adult responds with this behavior or sometimes any display of anger or will, he or she will be punished by even greater injury. In order not to bring this mighty adult wrath down on our tiny beings, we train ourselves as children not to respond to injury with anger. The most efficient way to do this is to prevent the message from getting to the brain. The habit, once learned, is difficult to break.

But why is it so difficult, if it no longer serves us once we are grown? Nature, never one to waste energy undoing an adaptive trait unless she has to, is primarily interested in insuring that we live long enough to reproduce—in other words, that we make it through to adolescence. So she has given us the ability—in fact, the instinctive drive—to suppress any behavior that might get us killed, maimed, or otherwise deactivated during childhood. That this adaptive behavior can turn us into unhappy and often physically damaged adults is something with which she doesn't bother to concern herself—too much else to worry about. Or perhaps she figures that with all that intellect she's loaded into us, we'll figure it out sooner or later.

Of course, none of this was on my mind as I sought out a Reiki practitioner to continue the process of recovery that had started on Janice's living-room floor. I was interested in physical comfort and relief from pain, and that is exactly what I got. After six months of treatment, all my back pain was gone, and many memories of childhood suffering had come back to me. These impressive results inspired me to want to study Reiki technique, mostly in order to share it with my friends, but my practitioner discouraged me. In fact, she refused to recommend me for the training unless I were seriously interested in using it professionally, which I honestly told her I was not.

Reiki was not, in those days, nearly the widespread phenomenon it has become today, when Reiki practitioners are as plentiful as organic carrots. Only one person was doing Reiki training in the whole country, and access to her workshops was tightly controlled by those who had already studied it.

MACROBIOTICS AND MERIDIANS

A year later, in the summer of 1985, the Gilligans' only child, Patrick, was diagnosed with a brain tumor. It threw us all into a state of shock, and he was quickly swept up into the medical world of surgery and radiation. Michelle Clifton remembered reading a book about some kind of diet that had saved the life of a cancer patient, and I was soon in a bookstore, tracking down Anthony Satillero's *Recalled by Life.* Just beside it I noticed *The Cancer Prevention Diet,* by Michio Kushi and Alex Jack, and decided on impulse to buy that as well.

I read them both in two days and emerged from the glut of words and information hopeful, if a little stunned. Satillero's book recounted the story of his recovery from a near-fatal cancer, due to a chance encounter with some hitchhikers who turned him on to a strange diet consisting mostly of whole grains, vegetables, beans, something called miso soup, and (ugh, yes) seaweed! As an anesthesiologist and administrator at a major Philadelphia hospital, he was not at all temperamentally or intellectually inclined toward a dietary approach. But his scans had been getting worse and worse, his energy was failing, and he was desperate. He later returned to the health food store where he had dropped them off, to be inducted into the strange (and as it turned out, life-saving) practice of macrobiotics.

In Michio Kushi's book I read with horror all about what the great American diet (or my version of it, which inclined more heavily toward Diet Coke than Twinkies) was doing to my body and my emotional well-being.

Kushi puts forth the simple argument that cancer, like all forms of disease, represents an imbalance in the body. A tumor represents the body's attempt to limit the expression of that imbalance to one area, so the rest of the body can continue to function. The most effective way to heal is to restore balance, and the key to doing that is to have a diet that allows the body to function easily and efficiently, wasting no extra energy on getting rid of unnecessary, unnatural, and toxic substances.

Until that time I had blithely assumed that one of Nature's greatest miracles was the ability to take whatever I ate and magically turn it into more of me. My only concern, like that of so many American women, was that it sometimes made it into much more of me than I wanted to be carrying around. Now I was discovering that with almost every mouthful, I was slowly but surely shortening my life.

Never one to embrace half-measures, I threw myself into the rituals of macrobiotic cooking, starting with the recipes at the back of Kushi's book. I figured I could make myself do just about anything for three months, and at the end of that time, I could evaluate its effects and see if I wanted to continue. So after shelling out a couple hundred dollars for all the requisite equipment (pressure cooker, stainless steel pots and pans, really sharp knives, and sushi mats), I launched into a regime that seemed at first to fill up my life with shopping for food, washing food, cutting food, cooking food, *chewing* food (at least a hundred times each mouthful), washing dishes, and then going out to shop for food again.

Within three weeks I noticed some remarkable changes. For one, my lifelong insomnia had vanished. I, who hadn't slept soundly for two nights in a row since childhood, was putting my head down on the pillow and drifting off almost immediately for a solid eight hours, night after blissful night. My swimming time had improved, and all kinds of little aches and pains I had developed from weight training just disappeared. I could actually lower myself into the bathtub at the end of the day without creaking. Finally, my mood swings were gone—the ones that came along out of nowhere, with little voices urging me to step in front of a truck on a beautiful sunny day.

This was my first in-depth intellectual exposure to the world of oriental medicine and its concepts of energy—the energy of organs, the energy carried through the body in pathways called meridians, and the interactive energies of our environment, including the food we take from it and put into our bodies. I began reading books about acupuncture and gradually familiarized myself with its energy map of the body.

The acupuncture meridian system consists of twelve primary channels of energy (or qi, pronounced "chee") that, if you hold your arms above your head, run vertically through the body; six of them terminate in the hands and six in the feet. They energize twelve different organs, some of which are not recognized in Western medicine, and they seem to have a functional but not a physical reality in the body. They also energize the tissues through which they pass, and they influence and are influenced by the emotions. They come in pairs, which balance and complement each other. There is both constitutional qi, the energy we are born with, and conditional qi, the energy we bring into our body on a daily basis with what we eat and drink, how we breathe, how we think, how we feel, and the environment in which we place ourselves.

In time I came up with my own associations of organs and meridians with emotions, some of which corresponded with classical Chinese medical theory and some of which didn't. In Chinese medicine all the paired organs deal with different aspects of the same feeling. In my system they govern complementary but not identical feelings. By *complementary* I mean a feeling that can't be felt at the same time that you're feeling its complement. These are pain and anger, and love and fear. You cannot, at the same moment, experience pain and anger in your body. Pain carries you inward, toward the self, and anger moves you outward, toward others. The same is true of love and fear. You take in information with fear, and you flow out from yourself to connect to others with love.

The more I worked with energy, the less I followed formal

maps, like the acupuncture system, and just put my hands wherever they were drawn. In an emergency, however, it is useful to know how to quickly affect an organ without having to stop and feel your way into it.

My next level of involvement with energy came that spring when I found a flyer for Reiki training in my mailbox. I seized the opportunity, not knowing that this was to be the first of many, many trainings and workshops involving energy healing. By that fall I had bought a massage table and was trying out everything I was learning on my friends.

Mike and Sonja, after reading both Kushi's and Satillero's books, decided to put Patrick on a macrobiotic diet. They credit that step with keeping him alive for two years longer than the doctors had predicted he would survive. I occasionally did Reiki on him and succeeded in bringing up his blood counts after chemotherapy. In the end, however, the struggle to save this beautiful young man's life was a losing one. He died four and a half years after the initial diagnosis, having gone through surgery, radiation, and chemotherapy. His death changed all our lives, and his medical treatment deepened my own dissatisfaction with a purely technological approach to healing.

REIKI AND THE CHAKRAS

The training I did in Reiki had two essential elements. The first was learning where on the body to place my hands, what to sense, and when to move my hands to the next position. The second part involved a ceremony in which the Reiki master who was conducting the training "hooked us up," one at a time, to the universal energy source that supposedly gives the work its power.

When the Reiki master, through her touch and her intention "hooked me up" to the universal energy source, I felt as if lightning were moving through my body and into my hands. I

ORGANS AND MERIDIANS

Organ	Organ Paired with	Meridian Path	Physical Function in Chinese Medicine	Emotional Function in Chinese Medicine	Emotional Function in My System
Lung	Large intestine	Near the shoulder, below the collarbone, off rib cage, to lower outer corner of thumbnail	Breathing	Sorrow	Pain
Large intestine	Lung	Lower outer corner of index fingernail	Excretion	Sorrow	Anger
Stomach	Spleen	Under pupil of eye, just above bone ridge, to lower outer corner of nail of second toe	Digestion	Not specific	Anger
Spleen	Stomach	Lower outer edge of big toenail to center of root of tongue	Combines functions of spleen and pancreas; influences sexual energy	Not specific, but disharmony causes worry and indecision	Pain
Heart	Small intestine	Heart, across top of chest and down inside of arm, to inside tip of little finger	Controls blood flow and supervises other organs	Not specific, but said to be injured by "too much joy"	Anger
Small intestine	Heart	Outside tip of little finger near bottom of nail, along back of arm to back of shoulder, across shoulder, up neck to face, to just in front of ear	Digestion	Not specific	Pain

Bladder	Kidneys	Inner corner of eye, up over head, down back and back of leg, to outer corner of little toe, at bottom of nail	Urination	Fear	Love; old anger
Kidneys	Bladder	Middle of bottom of foot, just below ball of foot, along inner leg, up chest, to middle of lower edge of collarbone	Produces urine; holds sexual energy; controls health of bones and of hearing	Fear; deep grief	Fear; old pain
Pericardium	Triple heater	Between ribs, next to nipple, down inside of arm, to top of middle finger	Protects heart	Not specific	Love
Triple heater	Pericardium	Outer side of tip of ring finger, near bottom of nail, along back of arm, across shoulder, around ear, to outer edge of eyebrow	"Has a name but not shape"; heats and distributes fluid to upper, middle, and lower body	Not specific	Fear
Gallbladder	Liver	Outer edge of eye, around ear, up over skull to forehead, back down side of body, to outer edge of fourth toe	Stores and secretes bile	Anger	Pain
Liver	Gallbladder	Inner edge of big toe, near bottom of nail, across top of foot, along side of leg, up chest to middle of side of rib cage, between seventh and eighth rib	Produces bile for digestion; stores and regulates blood	Anger	Anger

now believe that no such technique is necessary to get in touch with the energetic healing power of one's hands. I've realized that it's there as soon you touch someone with the intention to heal, and most of my students experience the same thing. On the rare occasions when people do seem to need some kind of jump start, I suggest that they say to themselves, "Let my hands be heavy and filled with light." At the time, however, being "hooked up" was a very powerful device to convince me that I could, indeed, use my hands to remove pain, induce states of deep relaxation, and stimulate the body's ability to heal.

I took the training in the spring of 1986 and discovered that if I worked on myself before I fell asleep, I would wake up in a relaxed and pleasant mood rather than with the bolt of paranoia that usually seized me the moment my eyes were open. I also discovered that I could cure my own sore throats and colds if I got to them right at the beginning, and I did similar work on my friends. Many headaches also succumbed to the magic of the Reiki touch.

That summer, seeking a country refuge where I could follow my macrobiotic ways, I discovered Kripalu, a yoga center in the Berkshire Mountains. During the week that I chose, they were offering something called *energy balancing*. I signed up and for five hours a day on six consecutive days, I learned and practiced the energy healing techniques that are at the core of most of the work in this genre being done in the United States today. We passed energy to each other with our hands palm to palm; "scanned" each other's bodies, trying to sense, without touching, where a pain or physical problem might be; and felt the energy fields radiating out from each other's bodies, seven in number, each with a different emotional, physical, and spiritual quality. To our delight and amazement, all twenty-seven of us were able to do at least some of the exercises with ease.

It was at Kripalu that I was introduced to the concept of the chakras: seven spinning vortices of light that are supposed to lie along the spine and are at the heart of Ayurvedic medicine, the traditional medicine of the subcontinent of India. The first chakra is located at the perineum (between the anus and the genitals), the second between the navel and the pubic bone, the third at the solar plexus, the fourth in the middle of the sternum just over the thymus gland, the fifth at the throat, the sixth on the brow, and the seventh at the crown of the head.

Chakra is the Sanskrit word for "wheel." Thousands of years ago, because dissection was forbidden in the Hindu religion, yogis meditated and went inside their bodies with their minds instead of with knives and hands. What they saw on their inner field of vision, over and over again, were these seven centers of light, each with a slightly different pattern inside its circle, and each with a different color—all the colors of the rainbow, in fact, starting with red at the bottom and ending with violet at the top.

Since everybody seemed to see the same thing in meditation consistently, the yogis concluded that they had discovered the fundamental energy anatomy of the human body, much as opening the body physically and always finding the heart in the same place leads to the general conclusion that it is always, more or less, slightly to the left of the center of the chest, behind the sternum.

The system was later expanded to include 365 *nadis*—tiny centers of energy, most of which, as it turns out, lie along the pathways of the acupuncture meridians. Many Western energy healers, like myself, combine the acupuncture and chakra systems, assuming that energy comes into the body through the chakras and is distributed to the rest of the body along the acupuncture meridians. In Ayurvedic tradition each chakra governs the activities of an area of the body but also an area of mental, emotional, and spiritual life as well. Thus a problem with the first, or lowest, chakra could indicate problems with the legs or the large intestine, problems with physical survival (like losing one's job or one's home), or a general sense of not being grounded or earthbound.

THE CHAKRAS

Chakra	Color	Location	Endocrine Gland Associated With	Physical Function	Emotional and Spiritual Function
First (root)	Red	Perineum (between anus and genitals)	Adrenal glands	Legs and lower body	Survival
Second	Orange	Between pubic bone and navel	Ovaries, testes, prostate	Sexuality and liquid balance of body through excretion	Sense of self and creativity
Third	Yellow	Solar plexus	Pancreas	Digestion	Relation-ships with family of origin and obsessive relation-ships of all kinds; the will
Fourth (heart)	Green	Center of chest	Thymus gland	Heart and lungs, breathing, and immune system	Universal love and connection to nature
Fifth (throat)	Azure	Throat	Thyroid and parathyroid	Speaking and hearing	Speaking your truth; taking in loving feeling from others
Sixth	Indigo	Forehead	Pituitary	Vision and intellect	Psychic vision
Seventh (crown)	Violet or white	Just above top of head	Pineal	Biological time-keeping	Spirituality

I have never seen a chakra, although people have claimed to have seen mine. But I have sensed very strong energetic pulls and other sensations at the places they are supposed to be. Healthy chakras are constantly taking in energy from the surrounding environment, just as the lungs take in air and the mouth and stomach water and food. When a chakra is not healthy, it either leaks energy out of the body, or deflects it to some area other than the one it normally nourishes and governs.

TESTING THE CHAKRAS

There are two mechanical ways to evaluate chakra energy: one using a pendulum, and the other using a muscle-testing technique called *applied kinesiology,* which is also commonly used by chiropractors to test for allergies and organ weakness. I hold a pendulum (virtually any weight, suspended from a chain or a string) a few inches above the body, over the site of the chakra. If it swings in a large clockwise circle, the chakra is healthy. If it swings in a clockwise ellipse, the chakra is diverting its energy to other parts of the body, or to other issues. If it swings counterclockwise, the chakra is so weak, or so blocked, that it is allowing energy to leak out of the body. No one seems to know just why this is so, but I suspect that the answer lies in a concept in physics called nonconservation of parity, which tells us that there are always more neutrinos spinning in one direction than in another.

The muscle-testing technique, which is especially fun to use on large burly men, is more dramatic, but it gives information only about the strength or weakness of the chakra. I ask the patient to stand and hold one arm straight out beside him, parallel to the floor. Then I tell him to resist my attempts to push the arm back down to his side. When it is established that he can do this (indicating that we have located a strong muscle group), I ask him to place the opposite hand over each of his chakras in turn, while I repeat the experiment. Since most people who come to see me have some weakness in their emotional or physical health, there is always at least one chakra where resistance feels impossible. To their amazement, the raised arm collapses to their side when I push on it.

You can strengthen your own chakras with an exercise called *color breathing.* As you inhale, imagine yourself drawing light of the appropriate color for each chakra into its place along your spine—first red light into the perineum, then orange just below your navel, yellow at the solar plexus, green in the center of the chest, azure at the throat, indigo at the forehead, and violet or pure white, depending on your preference, at the crown. Imagine the cells in each are absorbing the light like little sponges, with every breath.

When I first started doing energy balancing work myself, I would do color breathing, then proceed to perform what is known as an *energy chelation,* a term and a practice originated by Roslyn Bruyere, the godmother of American energy healers. With a client lying supine on a massage table, I start with one palm at the sole of one foot and another wrapped around the ankle. I observe the energy, or lack of it, flowing between my hands, and I hold them there until I feel like moving them, which is when nothing more dynamic is happening. From there I move up the leg, ankle to knee and knee to groin, then repeat the sequence on the opposite leg. The first time I did this I was thrilled to feel energy start coursing between my hands, sometimes tingling, sometimes pulsing, sometimes very, very weak, but always there, and always growing stronger as I held my hands in a given position, until a kind of "energy plateau" was reached. When there is an energy deficiency or a block, I either feel nothing—a kind of blank, dead space between my hands— or I feel the energy running from one hand, across my shoulders, and down into the other hand, using my body as a channel instead of moving through the area I am holding on the patient's body. This is particularly common in knee injuries, when someone has cut off or blocked the energy of his anger, carried in the liver meridian, at the level of the knee, instead of allowing it to flow down the leg and into the big toe. After I keep my hands there for a while, I will start to feel a faint pulsing or tingling running from hand to hand, directly through the area I am holding. I know then that energy has started to move through the patient's body. When there is no alteration in this—no further increase in intensity—I move my hands to the next position.

When I finish with the legs, I move on to the chakras. I put one hand high up between the thighs, with the palm facing the perineum, and the other between the navel and the pubic bone. Then the lower hand moves up to where the higher one was, and that moves to the solar plexus. So I continue, moving on to the chest, the throat, and the forehead. I usually work on the crown chakra by standing at the patient's head with my hands touching at the wrists and fanning out from the center of his or her skull.

The Body Speaks

All those years ago at Kripalu, it was when I did a chelation with the first woman on whom I worked that I felt something different and strange for the first time. In the area of her second chakra, between her navel and her pubic bone, I felt, rather than saw, not just energy but something that I identified as gray and dense and somehow very sad. I felt it lighten and feel less dense under my touch, and she began to cry. At the end of the session, when I told her what I had experienced, she told me that she had had a hysterectomy and that there had been a lot of pain after the surgery. We both surmised that what I was feeling was the internal scar tissue.

A couple of days later I was partnered with an intense

young man in his late twenties. When I reached his fourth chakra—at the center of his chest, where the thymus gland is—my hand started to vibrate, and I got an image of a man yelling at a teenage boy. I somehow knew that this was his father, but I was at a loss about what to do with this information. Finally I said, "I see your father yelling at you," and he began to sob and groan. I knew that he was furious, and I would have loved to have him get up off the table and do one of the anger devices we used to do in group at just such moments, with the feeling so present in his body.

I realized, however, that this would be considered disruptive of everyone else's work. When the session was over, he told me, "I knew that this was going to happen." I decided to forge ahead and suggested that he might like to do an anger device, under my direction. He wouldn't. "I have my own way of dealing with this," he told me.

It was my experiences during this week at Kripalu—where something significant happened literally every time I touched someone and every time someone touched me—that brought me to consider healing as a profession. It also made me realize that there was a connection between the work I'd done in the encounter group and my own style of healing. From that time on, energy translated itself into emotional messages for me, and following these messages became the essence of my work as a healer.

The first person I worked on that fall was a neighbor with a back problem. When, in the course of the energy chelation, I put my hands at the front and back of his third chakra, at the level of his solar plexus, an image came to me of him as a little boy crouched and cowering in a corner of a room, with a woman standing over him. I shared this with him, only to realize from his utter lack of response that he had fallen asleep on the table.

When I was finished, I woke him up, and he told me that he was feeling so relaxed that his back no longer bothered him.

I did not share the image with him, thinking that perhaps he had his reasons for not wanting to be aware of the messages of his body, and that I should honor this. The next day he knocked on my door to tell me that he had slept eleven hours that night and had had a powerful dream about his mother that he felt was very liberating. He apologized for having fallen asleep on the table. "I think it was the Chinese food I ate just before I saw you," he said.

I subsequently noticed that people would often fall asleep not just on the table but during the meditations I led them through. It would invariably happen when my words or my hands reached a place in their bodies or in their histories where some trauma they were not ready to deal with was lurking.

As I have said, the process of getting messages about emotions from parts of the body I was touching became a regular part of my healing work. I could feel anger in an injured knee, or fear in a stiff neck. I often received images, words, numbers, and phrases as well. Numbers turned out to be the age at which the emotional or energetic underpinning of the problem had begun, words and phrases referred to the other people involved, and images were the initiating events. Eventually I would get these messages without even touching someone. They would start to describe a problem to me, or a situation in their life, and I would sense the part of the body holding the information about it and what the underlying emotion was. I could pinpoint from where in the body the feeling was emanating with great accuracy, and I was getting a great deal of additional information as well. Not with everybody and not all the time—but the more I worked, the better I was at it.

My first really intense experience of the power of this kind of healing occurred when a friend came to see me because a shoulder she had broken in a horseback-riding accident wasn't healing properly, and her doctors were concerned. Pale, blond, beautiful, and strikingly tall for a woman, at a little over six feet, Annabelle was given over to a kind of compulsive gaiety that seemed to lighten everybody's spirits but her own. When I put my hand on the injured shoulder, I had an image of a blond-haired child, around four or five, falling through the air. I asked her if she had ever fallen from a height when she was a little girl, and without answering she began to cry and make small, gasping sounds, like a child trying to catch her breath.

Finally her chest stopped heaving, and she spoke. "My—my—my father was an alcoholic," she said. "He was home one day looking after me. He put me on an open swing, and then he just went off—probably to get a drink. I remember swinging higher and higher, and then suddenly flying through the air toward the ground. I hurt myself very badly. In fact, although it didn't break, I fell on this shoulder," she said, slightly raising the one that she had recently broken. She then told me that she'd been riding with her father, on a vacation in Montana, when the recent accident occurred. A week later she called to tell me that she'd been to see the doctor again and that her shoulder had healed perfectly.

The healing that occurred for Annabelle came through a combination of energy and information. The energy that flowed through my hands into her body had allowed her body to feel safe enough to send me the image that contained the information about the underlying wound—probably the reason she had had the accident in the first place. When I gave her the information, the energy field around her—which I had activated by doing a chelation, starting with the legs and going through all the chakras—allowed her to feel safe enough to re-experience and release the ancient emotions about her father's neglect. When the horse threw her, her anger and her pain, held in the shoulder, had both called her to fall on just that spot and prevented healing from occurring until these feelings were attended to.

ANOTHER ACCIDENT, ANOTHER LIFE CHANGE

I was encouraged and intrigued by experiences like this one and by my almost hundred-percent success rate working with back pain, sore throats, and colds. But it wasn't until the spring of 1992, when I totaled my car in a head-on collision on a wet country road, that the full focus of my life shifted to healing.

Although the accident was not technically "my fault," I came to feel that it was my responsibility. That is to say, with the kind of New Agey slant on destiny that would have made me cringe a year earlier, I felt that I had brought it into my life to shock myself into making the kind of change that otherwise probably would not have occurred. My primary injury was a broken left collarbone, and it was just painful and disabling enough to make me feel weak, helpless, and dependent upon others much more intensely than I had been at any time since infancy.

A month after the accident, I took off for Boulder, for the second annual conference of the International Society for the Study of Subtle Energy and Energy Medicine. This group was founded by Elmer Green, a physicist at the Menninger Clinic who did a great deal of pioneering work in biofeedback. Its members are variously scientists, physicians, healers, and members of the public studying and interested in energy as it moves through and affects the human mind, body, and spirit. They call this human-related energy *subtle energy,* and they argue and debate quite a bit about its nature and activities. Some think it is generated by the body, and some think it creates the body, but they are all in agreement (in contrast, at the time, to the vast majority of the populace) that it exists.

This was the second such conference I had attended, and I knew that going there this time marked my commitment to take my healing work seriously, as a vital part of my being, which I had not done before. I was beginning to realize that healing was not just something that stimulated and intrigued me but something I couldn't live without.

I came back from the conference very excited about the people I had met and the things I had heard. The field of energy medicine and related subjects seemed to be coming into its own, and broad popular and professional acceptance of the relationship between energy and health lay just around the corner. This is just the kind of naïveté that has propelled me forward my entire life.

I wish I could say that I had the boldness at that time to abandon all else and just pursue my healing work. But I didn't. I had no confidence that I could support myself and was not eager to make the transition from the genteel poverty of documentary filmmaking to the utter economic uncertainty of a profession that few people had ever heard of and even fewer patronized.

I decided that my major contribution to healing would be to get a high-ranking health policy job and use my clout to introduce alternative medicine into public health policy. Since I knew nothing about the field, acquiring a degree in public health seemed a good way to start. Since all schools of public health were equal in their utter lack of interest in alternative medicine, I chose Columbia University's, which had the double advantage of being close to home and, because of my father's professorship in the astronomy department, tuition free.

I was at Columbia only a short time when I discovered that a center was forming to do research and to inform the public about alternative medicine. I called up the director and volunteered my services, which were gratefully accepted. A few months after I joined the Rosenthal Center, I was told that we'd gotten a call from someone in cardiothoracic surgery who was interested in setting up some kind of alternative medicine program for their patients. I was told to call him back to get the details.

I knew that the department of cardiothoracic surgery was

one of the few profit centers for the financially troubled Columbia Presbyterian Medical Center, and I hoped that they
would be prepared to fund some exciting new clinical initiative
with an impressive research component attached. When I finally
got to talk to the surgeon who had called, Mehmet Oz, I was
quickly disabused of this hope. He himself had been hoping
that the Rosenthal Center would have money for a program. I
quickly told Dr. Oz that we didn't. It was hard to tell which of
us was the more disappointed. I tried to think of a way to end
the conversation graciously so I could get back to answering the
calls and letters from the public that had been pouring into the
center.

"So what do you do?" Dr. Oz asked abruptly, perhaps sensing that he was about to lose me.

"Oh, I'm an energy healer," I said, half-hoping that this radical announcement would scare him away. "Um-hm," he said,
apparently waiting for more. "Well, I'm also a medical journal-
ist and a graduate student in public health, as well as a volunteer
at the Rosenthal Center."

"Would you be willing to come in for a meeting?"

Half of me said *Why bother?* and the other half was thinking that he had a hell of a lot more influence at the medical
center than we did, and was at least mildly interested in the
subject. Maybe we could parlay that interest into something
fundable. "I'd be delighted," I said, with what I hoped was convincing enthusiasm.

A week later I walked through the frosted-glass doors of the
department of cardiothoracic surgery, on the seventh floor of
the Milstein Pavilion, named for the New York real estate mag-
nate whose money built it and who sits on the hospital's board.
Thick carpeting, muted lighting, polished wood, leather furni-
ture, and tables piled with slick magazines made a stark contrast
with the sterility of the corridors just beyond, and an even
starker one with the streets below.

I was ushered into a small conference room in which several people seemed to have been waiting for my arrival. The purpose of the meeting, I discovered, was for me to present my ideas about what from the alternative medicine kit bag might be helpful to cardiac patients.

Having enjoyed many happy and healthy years on a macrobiotic diet, my first suggestion was that the hospital give the patients high-quality, organically grown vegetarian meals while they're there. The nutritionist was aghast. "I believe in a democratic approach," she told me. "I think patients should be allowed to eat what they want." This response ignores the fact that everybody ever surveyed on the question hates hospital food, and that long-term patients continually complain that their orders are frequently confused with other patients' or are just disregarded. It also ignores the mountain of data relating heart disease to diet. It does, however, explain why a few days after surgery, heart patients at Columbia (and many other hospitals) can be found eating waffles with butter and maple syrup for breakfast and roast beef with gravy for dinner.

To be perfectly fair to the nutritionist, the doctors were not far ahead of her on this point. Sometime later, as I continued to work with the department, a diabetic patient told me that his cardiologist had advised him that it was "all right to eat the cake—just stay away from the candy." I gave up temporarily, but when I started going into surgery and realized how important the kidneys and the liver are for cardiac survival, I started in again. Finally I drafted a memo entitled "From the Dinner Tray to the Operating Table," stressing the fact that we could be preparing our patients much better for surgery by giving them food that supports the functioning of those organs, and proposing a pilot program. My memo was sent off to the head of Food Services, but nothing happened. It was my first taste of bureaucratic defeat. Who would have to be convinced of what, I wondered, in order for things to change? It is a question I still find myself asking over and over.

At that first meeting on the seventh floor, having been shot down on the nutrition question, I moved ahead to suggest we try hypnosis. I had recently written an article for a health magazine about the use of preoperative hypnosis to improve postoperative recovery. There was a lot of data around on this, although almost everything written was in hypnosis journals, not in standard medical publications. More important, I knew that an experiment using hypnosis with cardiac surgical patients had been started but was never finished at another New York medical center. This meant that a protocol existed that had gotten through at least one hospital's institutional review board and therefore might get through Columbia's. (In every situation where "human subjects" are being experimented with and tested, the IRB must approve the experiment.)

Dr. Oz was not content with hypnosis. He wanted more suggestions. We talked a little about the problems that cardiac patients have, and he said he would like to focus on pain, stress, and depression. I agreed to meet the group again in a couple of weeks with a list of everything I could think of that could help these conditions.

The list I compiled was quite long—seventeen items in all, ranging from acupuncture and aromatherapy, to changing all the lighting in patients' rooms from fluorescent to incandescent, to cleaning the floors only with natural cleansers. I passed out the list to everyone at the next meeting. "Just get them to clean the rooms, Julie, and we'll be ahead of the game," the cardiac outreach woman leaned across the table and whispered to me.

Her remark underscored something that had bothered me ever since I walked through the glass doors of Milstein. Hospitals, I reasoned, should be about healing. Everyone who walks through their doors, for whatever reason, should feel healed by the experience. This should be as true for the people who work there as for the people who come there to be worked on, worked up, and worked over.

If it were happening, then getting the rooms cleaned (and getting well-cooked food to the right patients at the right time)

would not be an issue. There would be no sullenness and de-spair on the faces of the cleaning personnel, no cynicism and fa-tigue in the voices of the nurses, no terror on the faces of the medical students, and no arrogance oozing from the doctors. One night a couple of months later, I suggested to Dr. Oz on the phone that I run healing groups in which patients, doctors, nurses, administrators, and people who clean and cook for the patients get together as peers. "After all, everybody has some-thing that needs to be healed, and everybody has some kind of information which could help someone else."

"Maybe twenty years from now, when I have my own hos-pital," he replied. "But not now. Think of something else."

Dr. Oz finally decided to start a hypnosis experiment in which sixty first-time coronary bypass patients, randomly se-lected with matched controls, would be taught self-hypnosis be-fore their surgery. Jery Whitworth, the perfusionist, would do some of the instruction, and the rest would be done by an as-sistant of Dr. Oz, who was excited about the project. "That cov-ers a lot of our patients," Dr. Oz told me. "What are you going to do in the meantime?"

I stared at him blankly. "Well," I said after a pause, "I could do energy healing on your other patients. What have you got?"

"I have heart transplant, lung transplant, and artificial heart patients," he said. "But you can't say you're doing energy heal-ing."

"Okay. I'll say I'm doing 'energy evaluations.' " I was actu-ally somewhat relieved, since I had never worked on people whose organs had been ripped out and replaced, and I had no idea how effective I might be.

"Good," he said. "What is energy healing, anyway?"

"When you have the time, I'll show you."

Chapter Three

THE ENERGY
OF HEALING

My ideas about energy, emotions, the body, and healing are
based on my experience of working with many healing modalities and all kinds of patients, and my belief in the unity of science and a holographic universe. A couple of years after the
encounter groups ended, in the course of a discussion we were
having with my father, who is a theoretical physicist, Sonja
Gilligan had the insight that the four feelings she had identified
corresponded to the four basic forces in physics—in fact, that
they *were* these forces, being experienced on a human level in
some way that physicists and biologists had yet to understand.

The four basic forces in physics are electromagnetism, gravity, the nuclear force, and the weak force. Electromagnetism, the
force that, as light and electricity, governs observation and communication, corresponds to fear. Gravitation is anger, with its
accelerative power. The nuclear force is pain, with its power to
pull in toward the center. The weak force, the last to be discovered and to date the most mysterious, is active whenever neu-

trinos are released or absorbed, as in the hydrogen-helium reaction which fuels stars like our sun, sending billions of neutrinos out into space. It corresponds to love, the radiant feeling of creation and connection.

From the human perspective, this means that when you feel fear, you are experiencing electromagnetism; when you feel anger, you are experiencing gravitation, which Einstein demonstrated is indistinguishable from acceleration; when you feel pain, you are experiencing the nuclear force; and when you feel love, you are experiencing the weak force. Each respective force field in the body is intensified when you feel the particular emotion identified with it. The only explanation I have for this truly wondrous phenomenon is Nature's extraordinary efficiency. It seems totally reasonable to me that our behavior should be directly governed by the very forces that wheel planets, stars, and galaxies around, control their birth and death, and are responsible for the creation and organization of the universe itself.

I got absolutely nowhere discussing this with my father, who maintained (as most physicists and biologists still do) that electromagnetism is the only force whose activities count in living matter, because life is all a question of chemical reactions. He was impressed when I relieved a stiffness in his shoulder by holding one of his toes. "But surely, sweetheart," he remonstrated with me later, "what you call energy isn't what we talk about in physics."

"It is if you consider the classical definition of energy that physics offers us—the ability to do work," I said, as I led him into the university's astronomy library and pointed to one of the long leather couches. "Lie down on your back. I'm going to show you something." I suspended a pendulum over his second chakra, between the navel and the pubic bone. After a couple of seconds it started to swing in a broad clockwise circle. "Daddy, you can see that my hand isn't moving. And there's not a breath of air in the room. So where do you think the energy is coming from that's moving the pendulum?"

"I don't know," he said.

"It's coming from your body, and it can't be electromagnetic, because that wouldn't make something move in a circle." We agreed at that point to disagree, and I went looking other places for corroborative evidence to support my ideas.

ANGER AND GRAVITATION

I did collect some anecdotal evidence on the correlation between anger and gravitation at the very same subtle energy conference that had moved me along toward my current path. At a panel on "anomalous medical phenomena," an orthopedic surgeon, who was doing more massage than surgery, posed the following problem. Very often, he had noticed, when his patients first got on the massage table, they seemed so heavy that he could barely slide his hand between them and the table. By the end of the session, by contrast, they seemed much lighter. He was so intrigued by this that he decided to weigh one of his patients, before and after the treatment. She had lost three pounds, which she subsequently regained over the next three days. Did anyone have an explanation for this? he wanted to know.

During the question period I proposed that when he massaged his patients, he was actually releasing anger from their bodies (a major factor in back pain, which is what he was treating them for) and thereby reducing their gravitational fields.

The normal emotional response to physical pain is anger. Conversely, anger held in the body creates an overload of energy that is felt as physical pain. When I worked on Annabelle's shoulder, I was releasing her ancient anger at her father for abandoning her, both relieving the shoulder's pain and allowing it to heal. My own shoulder felt lighter after Janice worked on me, as if there were now more space between the cells. Part of what she released was my anger at my mother for hitting me.

Further evidence of the relationship between anger and

gravitation is in the phenomenon of depression. It is now commonly accepted that depression is anger turned inward, against the self. The very quality of depression is both a mental and physical heaviness. Depressed people feel "weighed down." They can barely drag themselves around. This internalized anger increases their gravitational field, making it literally more difficult for them to move.

For more than twenty years I lived with this idea of forces and feelings, sporadically and always unsuccessfully trying to engage the interest of physicists and making a few desperate attempts to teach myself quantum mechanics without the benefit of any higher mathematics. When I began doing healing work, however, the idea that each force literally takes over the body and dominates it as we move from feeling state to feeling state came into focus. It is precisely this correlation that enables us to understand the forces of physics as we do, and why we find the laws that govern them of such compelling interest. The greatest physicist of our time, Albert Einstein, used to say that he "felt physics in his bones." I believe what he meant by this is that the truths of his body perfectly reflected the basic truths of the universe, and that he could sense in his physical being the correctness of a physical law.

TIME, LOVE, AND THE WEAK FORCE

The more healing I did, the more I thought about what healing energy is. I was convinced, as a lover of science and just plain common sense, that it wasn't anything mystical, involving angels, spirits, or other dimensions of reality.

If physical pain is anger, and tightness or stiffness is fear, I asked myself, then what is the healing energy that releases those conditions? One day it came to me that you have to love someone in order to heal him, and that that loving feeling itself is the primary healing energy. In terms of physics, love is associated with the weak force, the force released deep inside stars like the sun, where they create the energy that keeps us all alive. This mysterious weak force is the healing force.

If the weak force is the force that heals, what happens when I, as a healer, allow energy to stream through my hands into a patient? The particles released by the weak force are neutrinos. I imagine that streams of neutrinos, perhaps coherent streams like those produced by a laser, flow into the energy field and body of the patient, interacting with both. While it is usually maintained that neutrinos pass through matter without affecting it, I would insist on just the opposite: that they affect living matter in a way that we have yet to comprehend.

Consider the concert of love as healing energy. Everybody knows the feeling of love—of total acceptance of the self and everything around you. When love is focused on another person, it is the overwhelming desire for that person's happiness and well-being. It is the paramount state of nonjudgment. It also has a primitive, formless, undefended quality to it—and this is the state to which we must return, over and over again, if we are to heal.

Robert Becker, one of the pioneers of energy medicine, discovered that salamanders regenerate an amputated limb when the cells at the end of the stump dedifferentiate, then grow into all the various tissue cells needed to build a limb. Similarly he discovered that bone regenerates by having marrow cells dedifferentiate and reform as bone cells. This process of going back to a simpler, less defined, less defended state is at the essence of healing—and this state is the state of loving feeling.

It is also the postorgasmic state and the creative energy of the orgasm itself, as Wilhelm Reich correctly realized. Reich even desperately sought an interview with Einstein to try to convince him of the universal nature of this energy. Unfortunately he did not have the background in physics to make a convincing argument. That children and stars are created with the same energy was something that even the discoverer of relativity was not ready to accept.

Some Taoist texts use sexual energy, an intense form of loving feeling, in very specific exercises to heal different parts of the body. Special positions for intercourse are even prescribed for healing the ailments of either partner. When I mentioned this idea that love, and therefore sexual energy, is the energy of healing, to another healer, she came up with the insight that this must be the reason that it is very difficult to heal sexual abuse—the very energy that is the energy of healing has been distorted and wounded.

In an actual healing session, the love I feel for the patient—not because of any special virtue or spiritual quality on my part but because their vulnerability irresistibly draws love out of me—creates a safe space, or a vibrational environment, in which I can feel their feelings more clearly. It also releases my own intelligence and allows me to make connections that guide them informationally as well as energetically.

Sonja had an intuitive sense that love is also time, and after that initial discussion with my father, this set us off exploring another set of equivalencies between the world of feelings and the world of physics. Space, it seemed to us, has to correspond to fear: open, receptive, and the medium through which communication travels. Matter is pain, because of that feeling's relationship to information. Pain brings you to a place of knowing, and information exists in bits of matter. And energy has to be anger because the essence of anger is movement, and the most immediate effect of getting in touch with your anger is of being highly energized.

When I thought about love as the healing force, I thought about the power of time to heal—our sense that very often the process of life itself, moving us through time, or, if you will, moving time through us, brings us to a place of healing. Love is time, the great container in which everything else occurs. When we feel that we are running out of time, our panic is really about the false sense that we do not have enough love to sustain us.

Love is a feeling of the body. It grounds us in the body and its creative powers. People who suffer from serious disease have actually withdrawn both their love and their awareness from parts of their bodies, and the disease is, in part, a call to them to return to their physical beings in a much more attentive way. This attentiveness, in turn, can lead them to discover the secret history of wounds that the body holds so lovingly for them.

COMING INTO THE BODY

My own journey into healing has been a journey into my body, an attempt to inhabit it more completely. My original escape from the body had been through intense intellectualism and bulimia. But gradually I returned from the world of the intellect to the world of emotions, which bridges the brain to the body. I reconnected thought and feeling and admitted that the love I had taken in was what had made me smart.

In my early energy work, I experienced the flow of life's forces moving through me, forces which I gradually came to realize were the four emotions as I had learned to know them in the encounter group. Finally, I began to anchor my experience and understanding of these energies in organs, tissues, fluids, and cells.

As I learned more about breathing and movement, I discovered that I could bring my consciousness, my awareness, to any part of my physical being, large or small. My way of doing this is to say to myself, "Be your back; be your knee; etc." When I do this, I know that I am in touch with the part I have named, because I experience a definite shift in self-awareness, a different sense of internal space, of balance, quality of movement and ease of movement, vision, hearing, and often emotion as well.

How does this shift take place? There are two possible ways. The first is through a transmission of matter waves, whose existence de Broglie posited, which can be read and interpreted by the brain. The second way is through energetic communications that are going back and forth between cells and molecules within cells all the time. Such communications enable these billions of independent operators to collaborate as part of the vast bureaucracy called the body, in recognizable patterns, of organ, tissue, and fluid, which the brain, when directed to do so, can understand.

So much for being present with a part or subpart of the body. What does it mean to move from, breathe from, look from, or even listen from that body part? It means that the organ, tissue, fluid, or cell has an awareness and an intention that participates in these acts, and that we can willfully allow that awareness and intention to dominate our experience of them.

This ability was first demonstrated to me in a workshop run by Bonnie Bainbridge Cohen, founder of the School for Body-Mind Centering and a great pioneer of somatic work. Bending over slowly from the waist and then straightening up again with a movement that seemed to float her spine back into an upright position, Bonnie told us that she was "bending over from the bones and straightening up from the nerves." When she did it a second time, I could feel those tissues in my own body recording her movement. Then she had us do the same movements in pairs. Bending over, after instructing myself to "be your bones," I could feel each vertebra giving in to the pull of gravity as I rolled my spine forward. "Be your nerves," I said before coming back to an upright position. As I had seen Bonnie do, I seemed to float up lightly, with no sensation of bone at all in my body, and my awareness much closer to the surface of the skin.

At another point the group was instructed to improvise movement from each of the four primary fluids of the body. These are:

1. Cerebrospinal fluid, which bathes the brain and the spinal cord.

2. Blood.

3. Lymph, which is the clear liquid that carries cells essential to the immune system and cleans and filters the blood.

4. Synovial fluid, which lubricates the joints.

Moving from the cerebrospinal fluid felt light and vertical. As I looked around me, I saw people reaching arms toward the ceiling and taking easy jumps. When we came into our blood, the difference was striking. I found that my movements became much more horizontal in their orientation and lower to the ground. A feeling of power and aggression pervaded the room. In a flash I saw that each fluid has a distinct emotional and energetic quality. Cerebrospinal fluid carries the energy of fear and electromagnetism, while blood carries the energy of anger and gravitation. Lymph, with its close relationship to blood, has the quality of pain and the nuclear force. It also carries cells whose job it is to continually make the distinction between self and nonself in the body, as part of the immune system. Autoimmune disorders, in which the body attacks its own cells as if they were enemies, is a lymphatic system malfunction. This left synovial fluid, clear and, like cerebrospinal fluid, not containing any cells, to carry the energy of love and the weak force. When I and the others in the room went there with our awareness and started to move, we rotated our joints like Balinese dancers, like the spiraling of a baby down the birth canal and the intertwining of strands of DNA.

Having now led a number of untrained groups through this exercise, I believe that this awareness can be available to anybody. In order to experience it, I suggest that you just stand quietly for a few moments with your eyes closed and think about the fluid bathing your spine. As you do so, you may become aware of a subtle pulsing sensation and a slight, rhythmic expansion and contraction along its length. Allow yourself to sink into the sense of a fluid column running up and down your spine. Then begin to move.

For blood, focus on the color red, and feel it streaming through your being. Let the color carry you into movement.

For lymph, say "Bring me to the fluid by which I know myself." Feel a force moving through the body, filtering and cleaning, and then move with that force.

For synovial fluid, be alive in your joints. Sense the possibility of infinite rotation, flexibility, and change. Then let it carry you forward.

From thinking about the energies of fluids, it was a natural step to think about tissue in similar terms.

I concluded that nerves, which govern perception and communication, carry fear; muscles, which govern movement, carry anger; bones, creating structure, hold memory and pain; and bone marrow, at the very core of the skeleton, regenerating our blood, carries love.

The total picture looks like this:

FEELINGS	FORCES	FUNDAMENTALS OF THE UNIVERSE	FLUIDS	TISSUES
Fear	Electro-magnetism	Space	Cerebro-spinal fluid	Nerves
Anger	Gravitation	Energy	Blood	Muscles
Pain	Nuclear force	Matter	Lymph	Bone
Love	Weak force	Time	Synovial fluid	Bone marrow

The emotional defenses are held in the tissues adjacent to the ones holding the feelings. When I put my awareness into any of these secondary tissues, I couldn't get to a clear emotion. Only its defensive form was available to me.

FEELINGS, DEFENSES, AND TISSUES			
FEELING — TISSUE		DEFENSE — TISSUE	
Fear — Nerves		Hate — Skin	
Anger — Muscle		Resentment — Fat	
Pain — Bone		Contempt — Tendons	
Love — Bone marrow		Joy — Ligaments	

HIDING EMOTIONS—CREATING DISEASE

In very sick patients, something even more radical is going on. Feelings are being held in tissues that are not meant to carry them. A lung patient, for example, was carrying fear in his blood instead of anger. This made the blood watchful instead of active, as it needed to be. My heart patients very often had sorrow in their blood, and the energy of this sorrow, passing through the heart over and over again, weakened it. When Bonnie told me that the blood programs the heart, this made total sense. It also taught me that, after transplant surgery, I had to enlist the help of the blood in telling the heart all about its new body, and telling the body all about the heart.

Another example of a relationship between the shifting of emotions and disease is osteoporosis. Women hide their anger (and inactivate it) by pulling its energy out of the muscle and down into the bone. The bone then feels as if its gravitational field has been increased, and it gives up tissue to become what it feels is its appropriate weight. Exercise helps prevent osteoporosis because it moves the anger back into the muscle. The bone no longer senses itself as too heavy, and it makes more tissue. The problem occurs far less in men because their expressions of anger and aggressiveness are more accepted in our society and are allowed more range of expression.

I am frequently asked by physicians (with obviously no feel-

Hands
of
Life

ing for irony) how I can "anthropomorphize" the body so. What they mean is, how can I assume that these communications are going on among organs, tissues, fluids, and even cells and parts of cells? My response is that, first of all, I don't believe that what we call "consciousness" is localized to the brain. Rather, personality and memory exist in every cell of our bodies. In regression work people who had no prior knowledge of embryology were accurately able to describe their own conception and early embryological development. Memory precedes the formation of the nervous system and must therefore exist on a cellular level.

Moreover, if communication did not exist within and among cells, tissues, fluids, and organs, then the vast bureaucracy of the body, with billions and billions of tiny parts, would never be able to collaborate to form a working organism. The brain couldn't possibly be directing all this activity, because most of it happens faster than neural impulses can travel. My work, in directing my attention and that of my patients to parts of their bodies, consists of tuning our brain's awareness into these communications—allowing it to listen in on these conversations and participate in them.

THE HOLOGRAPHY OF THE BODY

This brings me to another belief that heavily affects my practice. One day Bonnie described to a group of us her experiences with a young girl with serious kidney problems. Since, in Chinese medicine, the kidneys are a major energy source for the body (the Chinese picture them as two little feet, embedded in our backs, pushing us along through life), Bonnie decided that the girl's basic problem was an energy deficiency and that the place to work on this was in the mitochondria, which are the parts of the cell in which ATP, the source of the cell's energy, is produced. Bringing her awareness there inside the girl's cells, she taught the girl how to use her intention to increase mitochondria production.

The essential idea behind this approach is that whatever is happening on a macroscopic level in the body (in the kidneys, for example) is also happening on a microscopic level (in the mitochondria). So with heart patients I will sometimes bring them down to a level of cellular awareness through a breathing technique that synchronizes the breathing of their lungs with the respiration of their cells. I start by having them observe their breathing and notice that all they have to do to sustain it is to exhale and allow the next breath to come to them. They have no need to make an effort to breathe in. Then I tell them that, just like the lungs, the cells also breathe, taking in oxygen and giving off waste gases that are carried away by the blood. I allow my own awareness to go to that place of cellular breathing as I tell them to come into their cells and feel this very gentle but insistent rhythm of respiration.

Then I ask them to go inside their cells and feel what is going on in their transport proteins, which are the cells' circulatory system. I ask them to focus on making that movement fluid and rhythmical, which in turn helps stabilize blood pressure and heart rate.

This concept of a holographic relationship between gross and fine parts of the body will, I believe, eventually be found to hold true on the molecular, atomic, and subatomic level as well. At the risk of bringing the scorn of biophysicists down on my head, I predict that we will eventually discover that even an electron in a sick person's body behaves differently from an electron in a healthy person's body.

Chapter Four

HEARTS
AND LUNGS

After I had already started treating his patients, I finally convinced Mehmet Oz to lie down on his own examining table and let me show him what I did. It was a little difficult, because he refused to turn his beeper off, and he got up off the table twice to answer pages. He also kept asking me what I was doing, and so I tried to explain as I went along.

He told me, as he lay down, that nothing was bothering him except for a slight pain in his foot, which he had hurt playing soccer with his daughters. When I put my hands there, I could feel rage held in his leg. "What were you angry about over the weekend?" I asked.

"Nothing," he said. Then, after a pause: "I lost a patient and it really bothers me."

"That's why you hurt your foot," I said. "Try to let the pain come down into my hand, and let the anger move with it."

His energy was vibrant and strong in most parts of his body, but there was a deficiency in his chest. I mentioned the weakness. "I once had a respiratory problem when I was a kid. Now my mother is convinced that I have weak lungs. Every time she calls, she asks me about them."

When I put my hands on his head, I felt a warmth and a glow there and felt myself suffused with loving feeling. "There's a very sweet energy in your head just now," I said.

He smiled. "I was just thinking about the little ones—my girls. I was seeing them running on the grass." His beeper went off again, and I decided to end the session. "Thanks," he said. "That was really interesting."

I decided, based on this experience, to treat as many of his colleagues as possible. I set up appointments with the chief cardiologist on the transplant unit, the psychiatrist, the social worker, and a number of the transplant coordinators. When I announced this plan to him, Dr. Oz nodded approvingly. "There's just one other little problem, Julie," he said. "Referrals."

Referrals, he informed me, are the life blood of a surgical practice. For cardiac surgeons, referrals come from cardiologists, because patients with chest pains and shortness of breath do not usually come knocking at a surgeon's door. These referring cardiologists were probably not steeped in alternative medical lore. What would happen to Dr. Oz's referrals when they heard about what I was doing with his surgical patients?

I hit upon a plan. I told him that I would put on my public health student hat and conduct a survey of the department's top ten referring cardiologists. I would tell them that I was doing a paper about awareness of alternative therapies in the medical community, without revealing anything about my own activities. Most of the questions would probe their experience, knowledge, and opinions of alternative medicine. Then, way down near the bottom, I would insert the following question: If a major academic medical center were to incorporate alternative therapies in its treatment of cardiac surgical patients, would you be (a) more likely to refer patients there, (b) less likely to refer patients there, or (c) as likely as you are now?

This plan seemed like a safe way to bring any threatening prejudices to the surface, and so I began calling cardiologists and interviewing them. When I had finished, the results surprised me: Eight out of the ten said that a surgical department's use of alternative therapies would not affect their referral patterns. The two others actually said that they would be more likely to refer to a department that incorporated these techniques.

From the beginning my work with the cardiac patients went extremely well, particularly in alleviating depression and pain. For the first few weeks, two other healers were with me— Michelle Clifton and my cousin, Michael Rosenbaum. As our work at the medical center proceeded, Michelle discovered that she loved the patients and the work but hated the feeling in the hospital. Michael was consistently curious and enthusiastic.

The routine we developed had almost comic overtones. Dr. Oz would sweep into a patient's room, with me following close behind. Michael and Michelle waited outside the door. The patient would smile. They were always glad to see their surgeon, no matter whom he was toting along with him. "This is my colleague, Julie Motz," he would say. They would shift their eyes to me for a moment, notice that I was not wearing a white coat and probably wonder why I was the only person in the hospital, apart from the Orthodox Jews, wearing a hat. Dr. Oz would pause, looking for a way to describe what I was about to do. He would smile at the patient, who by now had stopped smiling, and continue, "She does . . . she, uh . . . she wants to . . ." He would clear his throat. "I'd like her to spend some time with you. Would that be all right?"

They would look up at this man who had either just saved their life or was about to save their life, and then they would look at me again, and notice that I looked harmless, perhaps even a little friendly. "Oh, yes," they would say. "That will be just fine."

Then he would sweep out of the room, his white coat flapping, and I would motion for Michelle and Michael to join me at the patient's side. "What are you going to do?" the patient usually asked—a question they were too shy or too nervous to put to their doctor. "Whatever we can to make you feel better." They always liked this idea. It occurred to me that most of the people they see in the course of their hospital stay don't concern themselves with this simple goal.

Before we started to work, I would touch the patient gently, holding their hand, putting my palm on their forehead, or letting my hands rest gently on the tops of their feet. "What was going on in your life when all this started happening?" I would ask.

Everyone had a story, which they shared with a great deal of feeling. Although I was clearly the first person who had asked them this, they showed neither surprise nor reluctance when I did. It's almost as if they had been waiting for someone to touch them in just this way and to ask just this question. Their stories were filled with loss and disappointment: close relatives dying, children in trouble. Often—too often—they had been just at the brink of a time when they could finally relax and enjoy themselves. Their sorrows, I later learned, went back to childhood and had never been fully acknowledged or expressed. They often found themselves weeping as they talked, and they would blame the medication. "I'm not usually like this," they would say. It became clear to me that although the onset of the problem seemed sudden, they had spent years wearing out their hearts.

I told them that we would be touching them gently and moving energy through their bodies to help them heal. I would start by holding their feet, while Michael and Michelle positioned themselves at other places they were drawn to. I hadn't worked with other healers before, and it was wonderfully comforting to have so much energy and support in the room.

I often used the technique of energy chelation, although the name could not have been more unfortunate when dealing with heart patients and cardiologists. In conventional medicine chelation is a process of blood cleansing, originally used to get heavy metals, especially lead, out of the body. For some years a small group of doctors, most of them internists, have touted chelation as an alternative to heart medication and such techniques as angioplasty for clearing out clogged arteries. Conventional cardiologists believe it is mere quackery that keeps patients from receiving the serious treatment they need.

With the patients at Columbia, most of whom were in bed, I generally used the pendulum technique to measure the strength and quality of chakra energy. At first I used a beautiful ornament carved out of pear wood, which I subsequently lost, and then any piece of jewelry I happened to be wearing. I did this less for my own diagnostic purposes than to give them some visual evidence of the existence of energy and to satisfy the demand from the doctors to come up with "something we can measure."

The Lost Heart

One of our first patients was Paul, a recent heart transplant. (Patients tend to become identified with, and identify themselves as, their surgeries.) He looked gaunt and tired, and his very worried wife explained to us that he had a pain in his leg, which was making it impossible for him to put in the time on the treadmill that his physical therapist had mandated for him. I explained to them both that we would be working to help boost his energy.

Paul looked so uncomfortable and so unhappy that I didn't bother with the pendulum or the formal steps of chelation. My first thought was simply to comfort him, and when I put my hands on his feet, he relaxed immediately. His wife also relaxed, her face softening out of its tension. Michael put his hand over Paul's heart, and Michelle took one of Paul's hands in hers. Michael said that he sensed the presence of the heart's donor and a lot of resistance to being in Paul's body. I moved to feel a point on the heart meridian, at the end of the little finger of Paul's right hand. It was utterly "flat," as if no energy were flowing through it at all. Holding the finger between two of my own, I touched a point on his chest, just above the heart, which is the other end of the meridian. His breathing deepened, and I felt energy starting to flow along the pathway between my hands.

There is as yet no clear scientific explanation for why inserting fine steel needles or simply touching points along a meridian will alter the quality of the energy moving between those points and affect the organ through which the meridian flows. I can't speak for the needles, but I have two theories that could possibly explain the phenomenon of touching. The first is *synchronous vibration*. It's a well-known phenomenon that if you put a number of grandfather clocks in the same room, eventually their pendulums will swing in synchronous periods with each other. Similarly, women who are very close emotionally and spend a great deal of time together often find that their menstrual periods occur at the same time. This has happened to me on a number of occasions. It may be that when I touch a patient, the energy of their body begins to align itself vibrationally with mine, and the meridian I am touching shifts. A similar synchronicity may occur with the energy of the acupuncturist who puts in the needles, but I've never seen a discussion of this.

The other possible explanation is that when I touch with a loving or a healing intent, that point of contact becomes a magnet for ambient energy in the room, which enters the person's body through my hand or finger at that point. In this theory I am actually attracting a flood of neutrinos that interact with other subatomic particles inside the body to alter the energy flow.

My next impulse was to put my hands over Paul's liver, which is frequently a factor in leg pain because the liver meridian runs down the inside of the leg, to the inner side of the big toe. This area felt very hot to the touch. When I mentioned this, Paul said that he had had pains there, as well as in his kidneys.

These pains were understandable from both a Western and an Eastern medical perspective. To prevent his body from rejecting the donor's heart, which it would normally perceive as a living foreign organism to be killed and gotten rid of, Paul was taking heavy doses of a variety of medications that would have been highly toxic to a healthy person. The heavy dose of anesthesia he had taken in the surgery was undoubtedly still in his system. These substances had to be metabolized in the liver and excreted through the kidneys. On an emotional level, the liver is thought to hold unexpressed anger, and the kidneys, deep sorrow and fear.

I put one hand on Paul's leg, where he felt the pain, and the other lower down, at the ankle. I explained to him that pain is often blocked energy that is being held very tightly in one part of the body. In Paul's case, the heat in his liver indicated that unexpressed anger was the cause of his energy block, but I didn't feel that he was ready for this information yet. I suggested that he expand the area of the pain, moving the energy down his leg toward my lower hand, letting more of his body be aware of it, and helping to dissipate it. He did this and told me that the pain was lessening.

Before leaving, I put my hand on Paul's forehead, right over the sixth chakra. A sudden sharp pain ran from the back of the base of my middle finger to my wrist. I knew, without knowing how, that this was his mother's rage, which he had been holding inside his head for her. When I mentioned it, his wife gave him an "I told you so" look.

A week later, when we entered Paul's room again, his wife greeted us warmly and introduced us to his daughter, who was visiting him. She told me that just after we left, the pain in his leg had subsided completely, and he was able to participate in his physical therapy regimen without any trouble. "The only problem," she said, drawing me out of his hearing range, "is that he's terribly depressed. He felt much better for a few hours after you saw him, but by the next day he was down again."

We worked on him again, doing a standard chelation and finishing with a beautiful meditation. Michael led Paul through it, having him visualize light coming into each part of his body, starting with his feet, while Michelle and I held the energy around him. Michael's voice has an extremely soothing quality, and he wove in images of love in the form of light coming into Paul from his wife, his daughter, our hands, and his new heart. His wife and daughter also went into trance as we worked, and they thanked us at the end for a very relaxing and moving experience. His daughter told us that a headache she had had all day had disappeared.

Driving home, I found myself wondering if Paul missed his old heart. Before studying oriental medicine, I never thought much about my organs. I just assumed that they were part of me, somehow all working together to run my body. I wasn't even sure of exactly where they were or what each of them did; nor did it seem terribly important to know these things. In fact, I felt more guilt about the fact that I drove a car without understanding the workings of the internal combustion engine than that I lived in a body with no true understanding of my gallbladder, liver, or spleen.

After I'd been studying for a while, though, my organs assumed an emotional and energetic as well as physiological reality for me. When I woke up in the morning, instead of just looking at my face in the mirror and scrutinizing my body for every inch of sag and ounce of fat, I would check in with my organs and see how they were doing. Regular conversation with all my vital parts never became a habit, but they did gradually acquire a reality and a significance that made my involvement with other people's insides seem quite natural.

The heart is the wise governor of the body. What would it feel like to lose that friendly overseer, as Paul had, and have to take on another?

"Paul," I said the next time we saw him, walking over to his bed and putting my hands on his feet, "I've been wondering. Do you miss your old heart?"

He took a deep breath and sighed. "No one has ever asked me that," he said. "And nobody knows what it's like. Of course I do." Suddenly he was sobbing.

"Paul, we're going to do a little ceremony here to allow you to say good-bye to your heart. Just keep looking at me while I speak." Michael once more put his hand over Paul's heart, and Michelle held the little finger of his left hand on either side of the nail, stimulating both the heart meridian and the meridian of its paired organ, the small intestine. I remembered the resistance Michael had felt the last time, and wondered if it was the energy of Paul's old heart, holding the new heart at bay.

"I want you to start to say good-bye to your old heart and to release it with love. I want you to know that if there is a heaven for hearts, yours has certainly gone there. I want you to let it go, like an old friend who is leaving your life to make way for another. I want you to thank it for keeping you alive all these years, and for hanging on so staunchly at the end, sustaining your life until a new heart came along. Thank it for protecting all the people you loved, and for carrying you forward toward what you desired. Thank it for giving up its life, so that the rest of your body could live and continue in this world, making a home for your spirit until the spirit itself is ready to leave. And promise it that your new heart will protect all the people it loved, and fight for all the things it believed in.

"Now I want you to talk to your new heart and welcome it into your body. Tell it that you are just as excited about its information and its history as you hope it will be about yours. Tell it that you intend to honor and to use everything it knows. And know, Paul, that you are giving this heart a life that it would never have had without you."

I realized from the look of relief on Paul's face, as I spoke the last sentence, that a terrible burden of guilt had been removed—the guilt that someone had had to die in order for him to live.

Michael said that he saw threads of light disengaging from the area of Paul's heart as I was speaking. I was drawn to work again on his kidneys, which were giving off a great deal of heat, and at his throat, which felt blocked. "You must allow yourself to be heard, Paul," I told him. "Your new heart will give you the energy to speak up. Don't disappoint it!"

When we returned the following week, Paul's depression was gone, and he smiled as we entered the room. "He has two marriages now," his wife told me. "He's married to me and to his heart."

DISTANT HEALING

My next experience with a transplant patient came a couple of weeks later. Dr. Oz handed me a list with the names and room numbers of patients he would like us to see. Then he grabbed it back and scratched one off. "I forgot," he said. "This guy's in isolation."

"What does that mean?" Michael asked.

"It means you can't touch him, and you shouldn't go into his room. Too bad. I just gave him a lung transplant, and he really needs help."

"What does he need?" I asked.

"What he needs is to bring up the oxygen levels in his blood."

"We could try, if we could see him," I said. "How long will he be in isolation?"

"We don't have to see him," Michael said.

"We don't?"

"We could do a distant healing."

Never having done or experienced one before, I stared at Michael blankly. His attitude was so positive, however, that I was dazzled into thinking it might be possible. "Okay," I said, "we'll give it a try."

Michael and I walked past the isolated patient's room to a drab little space with plastic-covered chairs at the end of the corridor, euphemistically dubbed the "solarium." We sat down opposite each other and closed our eyes. I relaxed and allowed my awareness to enter Thomas's body—and was amazed at how much information came flooding into me. His gravitational field seemed to be pulled to the very back of his body, which told me that he was withholding anger. Energetically—which is to say, with my intention—I moved it forward. Then I sent him the message "Be your blood." I felt fear in his blood and told him to move the fear into his cerebrospinal fluid, where it belonged. The blood then felt very free and sensuous in its movement. I told him to oxygenate his blood but got the message back that he was afraid of sending blood down into his genitals—in fact, he was afraid of his sexuality, which he anticipated would bring him pain. I moved the blood there with the message that it was safe to experience his genitals as an area of power.

In my imagination I put my hand on Thomas's head (actually holding it out in front of me and cupping the air) and felt a charge of sexual energy come into it. Then I put my hands out as if they were touching his chest and said, "I am here to feel you." Again there was an energy surge, but without the sexual feeling. I finished by doing the same with his hips, saying, "I am here to know you," and again the energy came rushing into my outstretched hands.

Comparing notes with Michael, I found that he had experienced a kind of vacancy in Thomas's right lung, then a sharp pain and a tightness in the chest. He also got the message that Thomas had been frightened by his father's anger and abused by him. He worked energetically to rebuild the lung and open the air sacs. On the left side he felt a constriction that he associated with Thomas's mother's fear, very tightly held in. With his intention he sent energy there, and after a while the lung seemed to feel safe enough to take in the energy and make more oxygen available to the blood.

The next week, we got to meet Thomas face to face, and I asked my usual question about life events around the onset of his problem. "My wife had just left me," he told us with great sadness. "She walked out on me and the kids. And then this thing happened. There is a positive side to it, though. If I hadn't gotten sick and gone on disability, I wouldn't have been able to stay home and take care of them. That was two years ago. I've been afraid to get involved with anybody since then. I haven't even dated. But I was just thinking the other day that it might be time for me to try to meet someone."

Later, Dr. Oz asked us if we had had a chance to work on Thomas again. "I don't know what you guys did," he said, "but his oxygen levels came right up that afternoon, and we took him out of isolation the next day."

Chapter Five

SURGICAL
JOURNEYS

While continuing to work on patients, I proceeded with my plans to neutralize potential departmental opposition by working on the staff members as well.

Michael and Michelle worked with me on most of the staff healings, and after a couple of weeks, when word got out about how relaxing and revivifying the work was, we were flooded with requests. One of the first people we worked on was Donna Mancini, the chief cardiologist with the transplant unit and an extremely dedicated physician with a strong personal commitment to her patients, who universally adored her.

Petite and soft-spoken, she lay down on the examining table in the room we had commandeered, while we positioned ourselves around her to do a chelation. When I put my hand over her fifth chakra, at the center of her neck, I felt what I would later call the "doctor's throat." Michael, who also sensed a block there, told me that it indicated both cold hands and feet, which

Dr. Mancini confirmed that she had. Michael also said that it connoted difficulty taking in feeling from other people.

"Donna," I said, holding my hands very lightly at the front and back of her neck, "you spend all your time pouring feeling and concern into your patients. They love you for it. You have to relax this part of your body and let that feeling come back into you." Then, remembering that the throat chakra also governs hearing, I said, "You have to listen for their love and take in their words." I felt the tension dissolve, and Michael, standing at her feet, felt the energy start to flow down her body.

When I saw Dr. Oz the next week, he said, "You know, you really had an effect on Donna. Usually we can hardly hear her in our meetings. But for two days after you worked on her, this tiny woman had this huge booming voice." He also told me how pleased he was with the work we'd done on the nurses who were the transplant coordinators. "They're really burned out, and they really need something like this," he said.

Words from the Heart

Eventually Michael and Michelle stopped working with me as their own professional lives made more demands on their time. After they left, I missed the warmth of their company, their insights, their wonderful healing energy, and the insulation that their support provided against the indifferent and often hostile hospital atmosphere. This hostility wasn't in any way directed against me; in fact, most of the nurses and orderlies on the floor were friendly and helpful, especially after I started a group to teach them energy healing techniques. It was just the general ambience of the place—a sterility that had nothing to do with guarding against bacteria and everything to do with guarding against feeling.

As the weeks went by, my one-time encounters with people in extreme states of emotional and physical depletion were increasingly distressing, especially now that Michelle and Michael were no longer working with me. I saw in each face, and felt in each body, how much healing needed to be done. As I came out of their rooms, my own heart sank, no matter how ecstatic I had felt while working with them. The emotional connection vanished in the sterility, indifference, and hostility of the corridors. This hospital was not a place where connections between people were treasured.

Later, I came to question my own reasons for being there at all. Why did I have to be the outsider, struggling to wrest responsiveness out of a huge, unwieldy bureaucracy? My work was creative and collaborative and was inevitably in tension with a structure that was mechanistic and hierarchical. Although as individuals many of the staff tried to make an emotional connection with the patients, in the end culture and politics were stronger than personality and morality.

I decided to concentrate on the LVAD patients because, unlike the other patients, they tended to stay in the hospital for an extended period of time, allowing for some continuity of treatment. After I did George's surgery, I turned my attention to the other four LVADs in the hospital. By the end of the month, hearts arrived for all of them.

The next surgery I worked on was Arthur's. He had pretty much isolated himself from the other patients, as if they had nothing to offer him, and spent most of his waking hours working on his laptop computer or issuing orders to unseen employees in his Michigan office over the phone. He seemed short-tempered and imperious. In our work together before the surgery, however, his facade of aloofness dissolved, and a small frightened child emerged. He was one of those people for whom the helplessness of being a surgical patient is initially terrifying but who then experience a powerful longing to be taken care of and a despair that it will never happen. I felt flattered when he told me that he looked forward to our sessions to-gether.

Arthur's surgery was another middle-of-the-night call, but I got into scrubs in time to walk along beside the gurney as he was wheeled into the elevator and taken down to the fourth-floor operating rooms for cardiac and neurosurgery. Like George, he kept saying how calm he was, but he was actually extremely nervous. He went under the anesthetic easily, and be-fore he was draped and the sterile field created, I had time to send energy to his kidneys and to his pericardium by touching points on his feet and hands. There was something alarmingly brutal about the way the surgical resident swabbed down the body, almost prodding it with the sponge at the end of the stick. He was so rough with the Foley catheter, which goes into the urethra to evacuate urine during the surgery, that blood started to spurt out. I noticed later, however, that he was extremely ten-der when working inside the body. Had something about the naked inert form frightened him? I wondered. Dr. Oz, by con-trast, stroked and patted the body gently, almost with reverence, as he laid down the sterile blue cloths. Later, when I asked him about his manner, he told me that he was trying to bond with the patient.

As Dr. Oz made the incision along the sternum, I leaned over and told Arthur to relax and feel the surgeon's love enter-ing his body. I found myself, as I had done with George, some-times whispering instructions or words of understanding and support directly into his ear, and sometimes just sending the message psychically, following my instinct about which kind of communication would be most effective each time. Through-out the surgery I felt waves of sorrow welling up in his chest. He was bleeding a great deal, and this wasting of his own blood seemed to carry a great deal of sexual pain in it. He had told me that he was afraid his wife might leave him because of his illness, and I wondered if this fear reflected some wound in their relationship. I told him to be his capillaries and was overwhelmed with a feeling of chaos and uncontrolled hysteria. I told him to feel his anger and focus it in his blood. Somehow the bleeding seemed like weeping and I sensed that he was desperately trying to show his grief to Dr. Oz, whom he experienced as his father—or else to take revenge on him, because the excessive hemorrhaging was bringing Dr. Oz as close to distress as I had seen him.

When Arthur's heart was out of his chest, I felt in him a sense of abandonment, as if he were a lost child. I reached my arms down under his back to hold him physically and told him to fill the space in his chest with light and energy.

By this time people in the room seemed comfortable enough with both my presence and my activities that I could ignore Dr. Oz's prior interdictions against "waving my hands over the hearts." When the new heart came into the room, I slipped out from my position at Arthur's head and sidled over to the ice chest. Resting my hands lightly on top of it, I acknowledged the heart's fear of the unknown and its sorrow about the death of its old body. I told it that it was in a safe place and was going to an even safer one, and I instructed it to prepare itself for a new adventure.

Returning to Arthur, I found him frightened and uncertain about this new life coming into his body. (With hindsight, I now realize that this probably had something to do with his mother's feelings about her pregnancy with him. I discuss the role that prenatal memories play in the experience of surgery in Chapter 11.) I told him that his new heart would make it easier for him to take in love, because he would be able to protect it.

I felt energized and happy after the surgery, but the next day I had a headache, a sense of distress in my own chest, and needed to keep gasping large gulps of air. I resolved to watch my own breathing during surgery, and to ground myself more. I later learned from Roslyn Bruyere that under general anesthesia the energy field of a patient collects around the head, almost leaving the body. Thereafter I took care during surgery to ground the patient's field once he was under, placing my hands on his feet, his knees, and his groin and keeping them there until the energy flowed strongly under my touch.

Grounding the field in this way, I believe, allows the patient to be more present during the surgery, and the more present a patient is during surgery, the less trauma and postoperative pain there is likely to be. While it may seem contradictory to talk about someone being "present" who is, for all medical purposes, "unconscious," my own experiences have convinced me that not only do patients hear and take in verbally and psychically transmitted messages under anesthesia, but they also make decisions about just how present and conscious they want to be— and that this is often determined by what is going on in the operating room.

GOING UNCONSCIOUS

Although I worked mostly on LVAD transplant cases, occasionally Dr. Oz would ask me to work on a bypass surgery with a patient who was not in the hypnosis study group. Two such cases brought home to me the extent to which patients control their awareness under anesthesia.

One day at the hospital I was introduced to a reporter who, I was told, was interested in my work but didn't want to wait around for a heart to come in for one of the LVADs or to be awakened in the middle of the night (when most transplant surgery is done) to observe an operation. Dr. Oz asked me if I would work with him on his first case the next day, to give the reporter a chance to see what an energy healer does in an operating room. I protested that there was not much to see, but since I'd never actually worked during a bypass case, I was eager to do it.

The patient, Barbara, was a wan but cheerful woman in her

forties who had collapsed at her job one day and been rushed to an upstate hospital that identified the problem but could not ultimately solve it. The crisis was caused by a severe blockage of the coronary arteries. These vessels branch off the aorta and form a "corona" around the heart, carrying oxygenated blood there before it goes anywhere else in the body. It was these blocked arteries that would be "bypassed" with veins taken from Barbara's legs, and with her mammary artery, sewn into place around the sites of the blockage.

That afternoon I went to her hospital room to do a healing session on her, to prepare her for the next morning's surgery. Her husband stayed in the room as I worked, and I was particularly moved by his tenderness and his terror. I sensed that his life revolved around Barbara, and the felt possibility of losing her loomed over him with dread. My healing session on Barbara started with a meditation to bring the energizing image of light up through her body, starting with the feet. With my hands holding her feet so that my thumbs were on her soles, just at the center, under the ball of each foot, I told her that I was touching the point that in Chinese medicine is called Bubbling Spring, the starting point for the kidney meridian.

"Nature has constructed us so that every time we take a step, we take in energy from the earth through these points to energize our kidneys," I told her. "The kidneys are very important in Chinese medicine. They are thought of as two little feet nestled in our backs, pushing us along through life. Both Chinese and Western medicine recognize them as partners in the work of the heart. Now I want you to bring your awareness here, where my thumbs are, and imagine light and energy coming into your feet at these points. Imagine every cell filling up with light and energy, and the feet feeling physically lighter as they do so—so light, in fact, that they could just float off your body, into space."

I talked Barbara through bringing light and energy into her lower legs, her knees, her thighs, and up into her pelvis. We moved it into the organs of digestion. "Everything you eat is automatically transformed into light and energy," I told her. Then into the rib cage, the lungs, and the heart. "When you breathe, you breathe in not just air but light and energy as well. And every beat of your heart sends not just blood but light and energy coursing through your body to nourish all the cells." Across the shoulders, down the arms, and into her hands. "Feel it streaming out from your hands. Everything you touch, you touch with light and energy. And everything you reach out for, you bring to yourself with light and energy.

"Now bring the light and the energy up into your throat, and know that every word you speak is filled with it, so that each word is the most perfect expression of your thoughts, and each thought effortlessly finds its expression in your words."

When the energy was finally at the top of her head, I told her to feel it coming up and through the crown like a fountain, showering down around her, forming a cocoon of energetic protection around her. "This is actually your own energy field that is always with you," I told her. "We were just articulating it and allowing you to feel it consciously for the first time."

After the meditation I did a chelation, spending extra time around her pelvis, her solar plexus, and her throat, where the meditation had seemed to have trouble waking up the tissue.

Finally I put her into trance with my touch and took her step by step through the surgery. I prepared the veins that would be excised from her legs for the challenge of traveling up to the heart and handling the pulsing arterial blood. I thanked the veins that would be left behind for taking on the work of doing additional drainage and cleansing. I prepared the brain for the experience of anesthesia and the bypass machine. Finally I thanked the body for allowing the shock of the surgical invasion in the interest of healing, and I encouraged it to take in love with every touch of hand or implement. At the end the love of Barbara's husband filled the room, and I was moved to say, "If something as miraculous as this surgery can take place—

if someone can open your body without harming it, move its parts to places they have never been, and heal you—then anything is possible, and any change you wish to make in your life can be made."

Barbara opened her eyes after a few moments and sighed. "That's the first positive thing anyone has said to me about this surgery," she said. "Thank you." I then warned her that old traumatic memories might come up while she was under anesthesia. If they did, I told her, I would be there to help her move through them and release any emotions about them that she'd been holding on to.

The next morning we went into the operating room together. John Matthews, a medical student with an interest in alternative medicine and some experience with energy healing, would work with me. Once the surgery was started, John would stand at Barbara's feet and, under my direction, touch various acupuncture points to help energize key organs and strengthen the flow of energy running through her body. Between us, we would create an energy bridge for Barbara to lie on.

The anesthesiologist had a great deal of trouble putting in the IV lines, and Barbara squirmed in pain as I held her other hand. An image came to me of a child being hit by her father and terrorized by the pain. He also had trouble getting the Swan catheter in. Both John and I, when we later compared notes, felt that her heart was uncomfortable with the way it was placed.

Because four sites had to be bypassed, not only saphenous vein segments from the leg but also the mammary artery were going to be used. But there was not enough usable vein in the calf for three grafts, and Mike Gardocki, a physician's assistant who regularly worked with Dr. Oz, moved up Barbara's leg to take a segment from the thigh. As he made the incision, a shiver passed through my groin, and I felt a memory of sexual abuse moving through Barbara's consciousness, and terror escalating within her. I told her that her sexual energy was for her own pleasure and her own creativity now, and I invited her to let the terror move through her body and to have compassion for the child to whom these things happened. I told her that the men who were now touching her body were here to heal her, not to hurt her.

As Dr. Oz searched for the mammary artery, I felt rage welling up in the back of Barbara's chest. I wondered if he was jiggling the Swan catheter, causing further discomfort in her heart. I told her to roar the anger out of her chest and allow it to energize her body. She started to do this, and then suddenly I felt very drowsy, as if I were about to fall asleep. This had never happened to me before in surgery, and for a few minutes it completely confused me. Then I realized that Barbara had not only cut off her anger but had decided to become more unconscious under the anesthesia. Her energy felt fuzzy and unfocused. I sensed that this was not a good sign and that it was important for her to stay present. I told John to move his hands to the kidney points on the bottom of Barbara's feet, which would wake up her adrenals. At the same time I leaned over and said as emphatically as I could into her ear, "Come back here!" I felt her return with a rush, and I was suddenly alert and wide awake again. It then felt to me as if she were holding her anger up in her head. I told John to move his hands to the gallbladder points, on the fourth toe, whose meridian goes up to the temples. I felt the energy coming into my hands and Barbara's anger dropping back down into her chest.

"Your chest is wide open. Just roar it out into the room," I told her this time.

When Barbara came off the bypass machine, her heart went "afib," which is to say, it couldn't sustain a regular rhythm. Dr. Oz decided to put a pacemaker in, and I went into her heart and was caught up in a wave of distraught moaning and weeping. Somehow I knew that this was an acknowledgment of her father's unspoken pain, which she had been trying to alleviate by

Hands
of
Life

8 7

processing it with her body. I told her that I understood her impulse to do this, but it was time to release it and live her own life.

When the surgery was over, John told me that when he moved his hands to touch her kidney points, an image came to him of a 1960s automobile. "Would you ask her about the car when you see her?" he asked. I gave him a kind of "Are you serious?" look, but then I realized that I was the last person in the world who should be discounting this kind of information.

Still, when I walked into Barbara's room a few days later to do a postoperative session, I felt a little embarrassed about bringing it up. John, however, was at my elbow and hissed a final "Ask her about the car" into my ear as I approached Barbara's bed.

Before I could open my mouth, Barbara looked up at me and asked, "Did anything happen?" I stared at her quizzically, wondering what she meant. "You said I might experience things during the surgery, like old memories. Did anything come up?"

John looked at me meaningfully, and I decided to plow ahead. "Well, there was one point during the surgery when I felt that you were very angry, and John got a picture of an automobile," I said, leaving out the part about its being a 1960s model. "Did you ever hit anyone with a car?" I smiled to show how much of a joke I thought it all was—and hated myself for my cowardice. Barbara shook her head. "Were you ever hit by a car, or did anything traumatic ever happen to you concerning an automobile?" I asked, now feeling kind of bad for John.

"No," Barbara said, "nothing." She looked away for a moment, and then suddenly her face darkened. "Wait," she said. "There *was* something that happened. When I was eight years old, my family went for a picnic on a lake in Connecticut. At the end of the day, they all got in their cars and drove away— without me. I stood in the road, crying and screaming, but nobody heard me. It took them four hours to realize that I was missing, and to come back and get me." I did a quick calculation and figured that Barbara would have been eight in 1961, which made John's image of the car exactly right.

Barbara seemed to be recovering well, except that the incision in her thigh wasn't healing properly and was giving her some pain. As I put my hand there, I remembered what happened in surgery. It would be neither appropriate or necessarily effective, I realized, to bring up the memory of sexual trauma that had come to me when they excised the vein. "Barbara," I said instead, leaning over her, "I want you to feel all the love your husband has poured into your body, all these years. And I want you to feel that that love is making it safe for you to heal." She called me the next day to tell me that the pain was gone and the wound was healing normally.

If my experience with Barbara led me to suspect that patients control their own levels of consciousness under anesthesia, my next experience with a bypass patient confirmed it. Donald was a relative of a friend of Dr. Oz's, and I was flattered that the surgeon was so eager to have me work with him on the case.

Donald seemed calm about having the IVs put in, so I spent the first part of the prep time standing at his feet, sending energy into the liver and kidneys. I remarked to Dr. Oz that his liver energy was very strong and I didn't think he was going bleed very much (the liver controls the clotting factor in the blood), which turned out to be the case. Under anesthesia Donald experienced the predictable sorrow and despair when his chest was opened, but something else was going on. Suddenly there seemed to be nothing between my hands, in spite of the fact that they were gripping his temples. I registered that Donald had left his body. I focused myself on being as physically present as possible and pulled him back in. Again I felt his sense of loss and pain, but I told him to let it wash through his body. Then all of a sudden he was gone again, and that strange feeling of holding air between my hands was back.

The third time this happened, I knew something fairly serious was wrong, because Dr. Oz abandoned his usual ironic speaking style (as in "Go ahead, go ahead, do that—but do you want to talk to the widow?") for a more direct approach. He said to the surgical resident who was assisting him, "Just because you're in a lousy mood, don't take it out on me, and don't take it out on the patient." The resident's hands were deep inside Donald's chest. I tried to figure out what he'd been doing wrong. I didn't want to embarrass him by asking, but I tuned in to his feeling of bitterness and resentment and felt relieved that Dr. Oz had called him on it. I then returned to my efforts to bring Donald's energy back into his body, with only intermittent success. When Donald was off bypass, and the case was nearly over, my heart sank as I realized that Dr. Oz was going to leave before it was finished and allow the resident to close the chest.

Although closing the chest is usually the least critical part of the surgery, and one that attending cardiac surgeons often leave to the residents or physician's assistants, I had expected Dr. Oz at least to watch, considering his earlier remark about the resident's carelessness. Technically nothing went wrong, but the young man wielded the needles at the end of the steel closing wires as if they were harpoons, and when he pulled them together, he yanked the sides of the sternum toward one another as if he were going to rip the bone right out of the chest.

I went home feeling saddened and disappointed by the whole affair—and woke up in the middle of the night. "I know why he was leaving his body!" I said out loud. Cursing myself for not realizing the cause on the spot, I realized that it had been Donald's way of coping with the hostility the resident was pouring into his open chest. I thought again about Barbara and the uncomfortable Swan catheter. It made perfect sense. You come into an operating room bringing the surgeon and his staff the gift of your trust. And then when you are utterly helpless, they hurt you in some way that transgresses that trust. You have no way to defend yourself, and so you withdraw your consciousness from what is happening to you, much as children do when they are hurt or betrayed in a situation where they cannot escape or fight back.

Five days after the surgery, I got a call from Donald, telling me that he had terrible pains in his chest and no one could figure out why. (Severe chest pains rarely persist more than three days after bypass surgery.) I went to see him, feeling myself in a quandary. I could not tell him about what had happened in the operating room without getting thrown out of the hospital. I put my hands over the sutures running up the middle of his chest and told him to bring his awareness back to the time of the closing. I told him to feel the love that had come into his body at that time, in spite of anything else that might have been happening in the operating room. He began to sob, and I asked him what he was feeling. "My father," he said. "My father died of a heart attack. I miss him."

"Tell him that, Donald," I said, "and let the pain leave your chest. Take a deep breath and tell him."

"I miss you, Daddy," he said. His chest shifted and settled under my hands, as he repeated this over and over again. When he was finished, his face looked relaxed and young.

"How do you feel?" I asked.

"Better," he said shyly. "And the pain is gone." I left feeling satisfied, but still wishing I had been prescient enough in the operating room to protect him from the resident's hostility, keep him present, process this feeling during the surgery, and spare him the pain.

THE HEART REMEMBERS

My next LVAD transplant case after Arthur was Silas. He had been in the hospital since August, when the quintuple bypass done in June stopped working, and he underwent another surgery to have a battery-powered LVAD put into his body. A short, thin, dour-looking man in his late forties, he was deeply depressed the first time I came into his room, and whatever it was I wanted to do, he told me, he didn't have time for it.

Six weeks later, however, when he saw me walking by, he called to me to come in. In contrast to his earlier mood, he now seemed eager to try anything that might help with his recovery. Using a pendulum to check his chakras, I found a block, characteristic of all LVAD patients, in the sixth chakra, which is in the forehead, in the area of the pituitary gland. Since eyesight and intellect, the two functions normally associated with this chakra, did not seem to be problem areas for the LVAD patients, I had a hunch that the block indicated some imbalance in the pituitary gland itself. At one point I thought of suggesting to one of the cardiologists that because LVAD patients had so many problems that no one seemed able to predict, their pituitary function should be checked out: a hormonal imbalance might explain some of them. (The pituitary gland is the "master gland" of the body's hormonal system.) I would have a problem, however, justifying to a physician why he should order the test: "You see, when I hold a pendulum over the patient's forehead . . ." In addition to the credibility problem, there was also the fact that the hospital was already complaining that it was losing money on the LVADs because of the length of stay and multiple complications, and additional tests would be costly.

Michael was still working with me at the time, and while I did an energy chelation on Silas, he stood with his hands on Silas's head and asked him to imagine himself getting a new and vibrant heart that fit him perfectly. He then asked Silas to see himself a week after the surgery, walking through a field with his new heart, and feel that heart beating contentedly as his family surrounded him. When we checked the chakras again, both the sixth and the seventh, which had been blocked before we started, were now open. Silas looked happy and peaceful and asked if we would come back.

That was in October, and I worked with Silas every week

until his surgery in December, noticing each time more and more relaxation in his body, and the emergence of an ironic wit. He had, in fact, become a source of great comfort and cheer for the other patients. His sister, to whom he was very close and who visited the hospital every day, had been almost crazed with fear when he was first put on the device. Now she, too, had relaxed, although they both found the waiting to be draining.

The night of the surgery, I made it into the operating room just as the anesthesiologist was putting in the IVs. Silas was the calmest patient I had seen yet—so calm that I could relax and focus on sending energy through his right hand as the Swan was being put in. As he was going under, I told Silas to go off to someplace beautiful and trust the surgeon to do his work. I told him, however, to leave enough of his awareness in the operating room to make sure his liver worked to metabolize the anesthesia and keep his clotting factor high, and to make sure his kidneys worked to produce urine and take toxins out of his body.

The surgery proceeded uneventfully, and just before Silas went on bypass, Dr. Oz gave the usual order to the anesthesiologist to start sending heparin into the IV, keeping the blood passing through the machine from becoming sticky and clotting. As it went in, my own brain registered that this heparin was a primary factor in postpump depression. I could feel the anger in Silas's brain, that the blood coming into it had a different quality from what it was used to. I told Silas to instruct his brain that it was not in danger and that no action needed to be taken. All it had to do was observe the experience and record it.

(Later I did a body-mind exercise [contacting the mind of the body] in which I went through open heart surgery step by step, as if I myself were experiencing it. When my blood "left" my body to go through the bypass machine, it felt extremely nervous and uncomfortable. As an experiment, I tried sending my cerebrospinal fluid through instead. It seemed to enjoy the journey much more. In fact, it was excited. Perhaps this is because cerebrospinal fluid contains no cells, or simply because, carrying the energy of fear, excitement, and perception and being wedded to the nervous system, it is always hungering for new information. In the future, I would tell patients' blood to behave as if it were spinal fluid for as long as it was out of the body.)

During Silas's surgery, when his LVAD was taken out, a wonderful sense of relief washed through his abdomen. When his heart was excised, however, there was a sense of being a lost child, similar to what George and Arthur had felt. I made the same suggestion: that he fill the space with energy and light.

When I went over to the new heart, I felt both panic and rage coming from the ice chest. I asked the transplant coordinator how we got the heart, and she told me that the donor was a suicide victim, but that they had decided to withhold this information from Silas because it might unsettle his family. It then became clear to me that the heart was angry at the donor's brain for its decision to end his life. I got the message that it had fought about this with the brain and lost. I told the heart that it was coming into a loving place where its fear and anger would be honored, and it seemed to calm down.

When I returned to stand at Silas's head, I was torn. I sensed that it was important to tell him just what was going on with the heart and what it was so upset about. But since a decision had been made not to tell him about the way the donor died, I had to honor it, not even relaying the information to him under anesthesia. So I did not say, "Look, this heart comes from a man who killed himself, and it's worried that you might do the same thing. You have to reassure it that you will do nothing to purposefully end its life." Instead, I told Silas that the heart had been severely traumatized and that he would have to love it, honor its past, and make it feel safe.

Once inside the body, the heart felt curious, then appeared to relax. Apparently, however, it was not about to trust Silas's nervous system, and a pacemaker had to be put in to assure a regular rhythm.

Bleeding was excessive after the heart was put in, so I told Silas to "be his blood" and heat it up so it would clot. He succeeded, and I left the surgery feeling calm and energized. The surgery was a success, and Silas became one of our happiest patients. But it took him a while to get out of the ICU, and I couldn't get over the feeling that his heart was taking its time to decide just how safe its new home was.

The Healing Flow of Anger

My next surgical patient was Susan, one of our sickest LVADs, with a leg that caused her a great deal of pain. In spite of the fact that her raspy ex-smoker's voice had been reduced to a hoarse whisper by her LVAD implant surgery, she was indefatigably cheerful. She had been promised that whatever had happened to her vocal cords would be corrected when they put in her new heart.

A former day-care worker, the walls of her room were covered with cards from adoring children and appreciative parents. Although I fall in love with all my patients, with Susan it was instantaneous, and I was moved to write her a poem. She, in turn, was flatteringly grateful for the relaxation and the relief from pain that my work brought her.

Among her concerns was her fear that she might go back to smoking once she was out of the hospital. I decided to try to help.

"Where in your body do you feel the desire to smoke?" I asked. She pointed to the center of her upper chest, and I put my hand there. Immediately I felt sorrow sweeping up my arm and coming into my own lungs. I saw a little girl of four, sitting in a corner and weeping. "In Chinese medicine the lungs are the seat of sorrow," I told her. "When you smoke, you are bringing dry heat into that area, to evaporate the sorrow. I wouldn't dream of asking you to give up cigarettes, unless we can find another way of dealing with this feeling. I want you to breathe into the space under my hand." As she did so, she began to cry. "I got an image of you as a little girl, weeping," I said.

"My parents used to hit us—but you know, everybody hit their kids in those days," she said.

"Imagine if right now, someone two or three times your size, with a hand as big as your face, came along and whacked you. How would you feel?" I asked.

"I'd be furious. I'd kill them," she said.

"Do you think it felt any different when you were a kid?" I asked. "The only difference is, you couldn't run away and you couldn't fight back. And the sorrow of that—all the sympathy you were longing to feel for the little girl to whom this happened—has been held in your chest. When you begin to take her side and feel her sorrow, you won't need to smoke."

She smiled. "You always make me feel so relaxed," she said, and closed her eyes. Two weeks later, when she felt the craving coming back again, we did another energetic treatment on her chest, dipping into a deeper level of pain that involved her sense of separation from her father. I told her to let her husband's love come into her chest and dry up the pain. In her brief time out of the hospital (she returned after her transplant operation because of unrelated complications), she did not pick up a cigarette.

The fullness and looseness about Susan's body matched her personality. Her husband David, by contrast, seemed tight and neatly put together. He clearly adored her and was torn between wanting to trust the doctors and worrying about what they were doing with her. Seeing them together, it struck me how important it is to have someone besides the medical team watching over you if you are going to survive your hospital stay successfully.

When Dr. Oz made the initial incision for Susan's heart

transplant, I felt anger flaming in her chest, not in her muscles but in her bones, where it was weakening tissue. (I later learned that she had osteoporosis.) I told her to send her anger into the muscles instead, where it belonged. Similarly, her blood was filled with sadness and mourning, and I told her to send the pain into her lymph, where it would become part of history and memory.

When her chest was opened, I got the feeling of an angry little girl, flailing about, fighting many battles and losing them. Her anger seemed futile, accomplishing nothing. I encounter this phenomenon repeatedly in cardiac patients, even in type A's like Arthur. They may be full of resentment, snapping at people about every little thing, but their anger about the things that hurt them profoundly has long since turned into despair.

Just before Susan went on bypass, Dr. Oz asked me how she was doing. I'd been feeling worry and concern in her, and I told him that she needed permission to enjoy herself. As I said this, relief swept throughout her body, and I felt that she was pleased that he had asked. I then remembered what David had told me the second time I saw Susan: that she had just retired from the day-care center, and they had made plans to go traveling together and really enjoy themselves at last, when her heart started to fail.

When the new heart was brought into the room (later than expected, with the usual jokes about the transport team stopping somewhere for a pizza), I made my now habitual move of stepping back from the operating table and walking over to the ice chest. Putting my hands over it, I got an image of two women in a car at night, yelling and screaming at each other. "How did we get the heart?" I asked Dr. Oz.

"A car crash," he said. "The mother was driving, and the daughter was killed."

After the heart was put in Susan's chest and sewn in place, Dr. Oz tried to "wean" her from the bypass machine. But the heart would not beat. He tried the electric paddles, cursing because nothing happened—and then, realizing that they had not been plugged in, cursed even more. When they were plugged in, the shock wave they sent through her chest failed to jolt the heart into action.

Remembering the image that had come to me at the ice chest, I realized that the heart was afraid to get angry or show aggression in any way. It was afraid that anger would lead to death, as it did in the car, mirroring Susan's own fear that anger brings only punishment. As Dr. Oz ordered chemicals pumped into her to stimulate the heart, I told Susan that she had to be willing to get angry—and to give her heart permission to get angry too. I then did what I had resisted doing up to now, because it looks a little odd and I would have felt, quite frankly, embarrassed. But now I held my hand up in the air, above the sheet marking off the sterile field, and sent energy directly into Susan's new heart. "Give up despair, and let hope come into your chest," I told her. "Fight for what you want." I felt the heart perk up. Dr. Oz announced that it was beating regularly and she was out of danger. Later, as I was changing my clothes in the room where the bypass machines were kept, one of the perfusionists came up to me, an expression of wonder and disbelief on his face. "I don't know what you did in there," he said, "but I've never seen a heart come back so far or so fast." I felt as if I'd won the Nobel Prize.

Even more rewarding, though, was the moment I spent with Susan's husband. Shortly before the surgery was completed, I ducked out to the family waiting room, where friends and relatives sit, and often sleep, for restless hours, waiting for word that their loved one will be returned to them in some state of wholeness. I told David that Susan was going to be okay, and I spontaneously hugged him. His natural reserve melted against my chest, and I felt a love so strong, it almost knocked me over. I went back into the operating room brimming with the feeling, which effortlessly flowed into Susan's body from my hands.

Julie
Motz

Why Am I Here?

Kenneth was the last LVAD whose transplant surgery I worked on that month, and about three hours into it, the utter insanity of what I was doing seized me. I looked around at the surgeons, gowned, gloved, and masked, peering intently into Kenneth's open chest, their miniature miner's headlamps plugged into machines behind them, their Bovies smoking and sizzling as they burned into flesh. I looked at the monitors and the ultrasound machine. I looked at the anesthesia machine with its tubes of gas, its ventilation device, and its computer screen. I looked at the huge halogen lamps overhead and over at the bypass machine, with its tubing and its gauges, manned by the two perfusionists. My eyes swept over the scrub nurse, passing instruments; the circulating nurse, the link between the sterile field and everything else in the room; and the LVAD coordinator, and I thought, *This is crazy. What am I doing here?*

It was like waking from a dream inside somebody else's head. I didn't even think these surgeries, costing tens of thousands of dollars, should be done. I didn't think people should be allowed to get this sick! I didn't believe in any of this.

Then I realized that, in spite of my outrage, my chance of somehow halting the great march of battered bodies into open heart surgery was very slim. Thousands of people believed that they could be healed only by having someone saw open their chest and physically touch their heart, as they themselves could never do. Many other people, like the surgeons I'd been working with, liked cutting open chests and moving things around inside. These two groups of people were likely to be coming together for a long time. So long as they did, I thought to myself, there would be a place for an energy healer.

Why, then, was I there? In part, I was there to satisfy my own curiosity about the meaning of these complex encounters. In terms of basic personality types, I had noticed that most of Dr. Oz's male patients resembled his father, and most of his female patients were like his mother. I had known for a long time that the people I worked on presented to me problems of my own that I needed to confront. Was this also true of surgeons?

I was also interested in what you might call the ritual aspects of surgery. Prevention is not very dramatic, but surgery, a high drama of rescue, with all the ceremony surrounding it, obviously has deep meaning for our society, both for the rescued and for the rescuers. For the patients, did it mean that somebody was taking their ancient pain seriously at last?

Kenneth's new heart seemed unusually happy, and when I saw him a few days after surgery, an incredible brightness shone in his eyes, almost as if some other, much younger and more animated person were peering out from inside him. I later discovered that he had gotten the heart of a twenty-five-year-old girl, who, he speculated, had been into a much healthier lifestyle than his own. A former greasy-food addict, he now found himself mysteriously craving salads.

Although my vanity as a healer was greatly nourished by physical results, I was even more moved when patients told me how important my presence had been to them. Yet this work, for which I was not being paid, was eating up my time. I had a degree to finish. Dr. Oz had promised repeatedly to find a way to pay me, but the politics of the situation were clearly going to defeat him. I decided that I would cut back on my work in the operating room and start an energy healing group for patients as a way of compensating them for this.

In spite of my resolution, however, I found myself drawn into three LVAD implant surgeries just because I happened to be at the hospital when the cases were being done and Dr. Oz invited me to join him.

*Julie
Motz*

GHOST ORGANS

The first of these cases was Angela, a large cheerful woman in her early fifties from Brooklyn, with a long history of heart trouble. Both in figure and spirit she reminded me of Susan, and her husband, Gary, had the same compactness of build as David, although he was more outgoing and less taciturn.

Angela had been brought to the hospital three days before with a heart attack, and when Dr. Oz opened her chest, he found that organ greatly enlarged. She had seemed to me unusually calm, both before and during the surgery, although she squeezed my hand with unusual fierceness as the IVs went in. I prepped her brain for receiving the heparin-laden blood, but it seemed to despair once the bypass was started. I suddenly remembered the work of the French otolaryngologist, Alfred Tomatis, who discovered that the upper musical registers of a singing voice energize the brain. Tomatis worked with French munitions workers who had lost their hearing and with singers who had lost their voices. He restored both by playing to them music in which the notes in the lower registers had been filtered out. Eventually he realized that upper register tones correspond to the mother's voice as it sounds to the infant in utero. He then worked with autistic and dyslexic children, playing their mothers' voices back to them as they would have sounded in the womb. I began singing softly into Angela's ear, a song with made-up syllables, in a very high soft voice. I could feel her brain activity picking up.

Toward the end of the operation, Angela's lungs seemed very tight. An image came to me of her screaming and screaming and screaming, in grief and in rage. "It's all right," I told her. "It's safe here, and we hear you." The lungs relaxed.

Angela's surgery was done on a Friday, and Dr. Oz called me on Saturday to ask if I could go in and see her, saying that she had awakened asking for the "energy lady." I explained to him that I was an hour away and had plans that would be difficult to change. I suggested that I do some long-distance healing on her instead, recalling the success that Michael and I had had with Thomas. "Tell her to make sure she's lying down and by herself tomorrow morning at eleven," I told him. "And tell her I'll work on her for half an hour."

At eleven o'clock on Sunday I lay down on the couch in my living room and allowed my consciousness to slip into Angela's body. When I reached the heart, I encountered a heavy, crowded feeling. I got an image of a woman, who I assumed was Angela's mother, and of her heart occupying the space in Angela's chest. A shudder ran through me, and I was at a loss as to what to do. I moved through the rest of her body, carrying light and energy with me, then came back to her heart. The weight and the image were still there, but their meaning eluded me.

"Ah, the energy lady," Angela said as I walked into her room on Monday. I apologized for not being able to come in on Sunday and asked her about her experience of my long-distance work. "It must have been relaxing," she said, "because I fell asleep."

As I started the energy chelation, I asked, "Angela, did your mother have a difficult life?"

"She had a terrible life." She began to sniffle. "My father died when I was very young, and she struggled terribly to take care of us."

"I know this may sound strange," I said, "but when I worked on you long distance, I got the distinct feeling that you were carrying your mother's heart—or at least the weight of your mother's heart—inside your chest. Does this make any sense to you?"

"You know, my whole life, I've always felt I never had time to do anything for myself, any of the things I really wanted to do. I always thought that I was just lazy, that I couldn't organize my life. But I think now that it was my mother's heart, this weight inside me, that I've been carrying around for her. I was always focused on what she needed and how hard things were for her."

"Do you think you could let it go?" I asked, placing my hand over her heart and remembering how huge it was when Dr. Oz opened her chest. "Do you think you could just give it back to her?"

"Yes," she said with a deep sigh. "I'm ready. This has been going on long enough." I felt a lightness coming into her.

This idea of "ghost organs" reminded me of some of the experimental work I had done on my own, after taking some of Bonnie Cohen's workshops. As I've mentioned, Bonnie would have her participants originate movement from different tissues, fluids, and organs of the body. I decided to get quite specific with this approach—to try, for example, not just to move from my liver but to raise my right leg from that organ, or to turn in a certain way from it.

Bonnie feels that a curling-up movement, like a starfish pulling in all its limbs toward its middle, reflects the radial symmetry that fetuses and very young infants experience in their bodies. I was doing this movement one day to see how I had lived in my body when I was very young, when it occurred to me to try to make the movement from my left ovary. I'd always felt some kind of energy imbalance there; from my earliest days in Reiki, my left ovary was the one place on my body where I felt I wanted the practitioner to hold her hand forever. Reciprocally, any bodyworker or energy healer who ever touched me there felt something like a magnetic force, almost gluing their hands to my skin.

I said to myself, "Curl up from your left ovary"—and suddenly I found the movement very stiff and difficult to make. On a whim I said, "Curl up from Mother's left ovary." To my surprise, the movement was very free and easy. Perplexed by this paradox and wondering where the stiffness came from, I then instructed myself to do the movement from my father's left testicle. Again it was stiff and difficult, almost painful. I then got an image of my father as a young boy, with two older girls standing over him.

Could it be that my father had been sexually humiliated as a child and I carried a memory of this in my left reproductive side? Certainly the curling-up movement was one a boy would make to protect his genitals. Could there also be a connection between this and my own experience of early sexual abuse?

I realized that we carry inside our bodies complete knowledge of our parents' bodies and of how they moved. My experience with Angela's heart told me that children can take on the energy of a parent's organ so powerfully that its vibrations wear out their own. If a parent isn't clear about a feeling and carries it around like a secret burden, the feeling is passed on to the vulnerable body of the child. I felt instinctively that when other channels of communication and love are closed to them, children allow this to happen in order both to understand and to heal their parents. They carry their parents' unacknowledged emotional scars for them, trying to share and lessen the weight of the pain. It made me wonder just whose hearts my patients were trying to get rid of when they went in for their transplant surgeries.

I experimented with this idea of body haunting one afternoon in the energy healing group I had organized for the patients. I asked them to raise their right arm, first from their own heart, then from their mothers', and then from their fathers'. Everybody connected easily to the idea of moving a limb from an organ—or, if you will, allowing the character of that organ to express itself through movement—proving to me that it is not just people who flock to esoteric workshops who are capable of such sensibilities. Each group member had a very different experience of the range and quality of movement when it originated from their own organ and those of their parents. One patient said that she was afraid to try moving from her father's heart, because when she brought her awareness there, she felt herself swallowed up by a cold darkness.

Almost a year to the day after the LVAD had been put into Angela's body, her new heart arrived. But due to a failure of the beeper that I'd finally broken down and bought, I only found out about it halfway through her surgery. On my way to the ICU, I passed Dr. Oz on the fourth floor, and he told me that her surgery was in progress and that the LVAD coordinator had tried to call but couldn't get me. The former chief resident, the newest surgeon on the service, was finishing the job.

Cursing my misconnection with communications technology, I rushed into the operating suite, pulled off my clothes, pulled on some ludicrously large scrubs, grabbed a mask, a cap, and booties, and headed for the cardiac OR, where Angela's surgery was in progress. I got there and took up my position at her head, just as the new heart was being sewn in. As the last stitch was put in place, I felt, rather than saw or heard, something like the flutter of wings rising up from her chest, and I had the feeling that her mother's heart had left her body forever, at last.

A few days later, when I told her this, a little hesitantly, she nodded and smiled. "Something happened to me this summer," she said. "I saw my mother—my mother, who is dead. I saw her just as plainly as I'm seeing you now. I was in bed, and she came into the room, looked at me, and shook her head. She didn't say anything. She just shook her head, then turned around and left."

When Angela told me this, I appreciated how long and arduous an individual's struggle for independence from a parent can be. When Angela was a little girl, she had used her heart's energy to help sustain her mother, postponing her own desires and her own pleasure until doing so became a habit. Finally her heart had rebelled. But by failing her, it had actually tried to save her and give her back to herself. I believe that through our work together she came to understand this and was able to use the surgery as a fulcrum for emotional and spiritual as well as physical healing.

Hands
of
Life

Chapter Six

PATIENTS
AND DOCTORS

Angela and Gary were two of the most faithful attendees of the cardiac energy healing group, which ranged in size from four to fifteen, depending upon how many patients could be rounded up, how many friends and family members decided to join them, and what occasional medical students and healers dropped in. The patients were shy about sharing what they experienced in the group, even when I asked them directly. "Relaxing, it's very relaxing," most of them told me most of the time, no matter what the exercise had been.

I taught them some very basic and simple stuff, starting off by having them sense the energy in their hands by holding them against each other, palm to palm, and then slowly moving them apart until they could feel a kind of pulling that kept them from wanting to make the space between them any greater. "Just feel the shape of the energy between your hands," I said. "Push in on it a little, and then pull back again. You'll find it has a kind of elastic quality." They were as delighted as I had been the first time I felt what seemed like a soft globe of resistance in the space between my palms.

Next I had them work in pairs, palm to palm, and experiment with sending and receiving energy with each other. They ran energy out through their right hands and drew it in through the left, then reversed directions. They also experimented with both partners trying to send energy and then both trying to receive at the same time. I often ended with a meditation in which I directed them to draw energy into their bodies through their feet, from the core of the earth. This was very similar to the meditation I did with Barbara, the difference being that I started with a simple hypnotic suggestion and anchored the energy flow to the center of the earth.

GROUNDING THE HEART

"I want you to raise your eyes to the ceiling without tilting your heads, and allow your eyelids to close over them," I began. "Now allow yourself to feel very light and easy, as if you are floating down through the chair. As if you are made out of clouds, and the chair is made out of clouds. Now bring your attention to the bottom of your feet, resting lightly on the floor. I want you to feel as if roots are growing down from your feet into the floor, just for a few inches. Now feel them growing down just as long as you are tall. And now feel them going all the way down the basement of the building and through the soil to the rock below. Now through the rock all the way down to the molten core of the earth.

"Now feel the heat and the energy from the core of the earth traveling back up along those roots, all the way up through the seven floors of this building, through this floor, and into your feet. Feel your feet tingle and glow with this energy, connecting you to the very center of the earth." I would continue to guide them in moving the energy up through their bodies, out the top of their heads, and down around them in a protective shower of light.

The grounding and the connection to the earth that supports it are extremely important for cardiac patients, because they tend to carry their energy primarily in their upper bodies. Roslyn Bruyere has observed that most Americans do this, and it is one of the reasons that heart disease is so prevalent here.

The absence of an energetic connection through the lower body and the legs to the earth is one way of short-circuiting anger and rendering it impotent. It means, quite literally, that you can't push off from the ground and accelerate. Nor can you hold your ground, anchor yourself, and defend yourself from a stable position. If, as a child, you're intimidated out of showing and using your anger, you learn to protect yourself by automatically short-circuiting it.

My study of embryology taught me that fetal circulation is different in a number of important ways from circulation after birth. For one thing, respiration bypasses the lungs, and the fetus uses the mother's lungs for the important task of clearing waste gases out of the blood and replenishing it with oxygen. For another, the growing fetus gets all the nutrients it needs, in addition to oxygen, directly from the blood, so that respiration, ingestion, and digestion are joined in a single function; the umbilical cord serves as both trachea and esophagus. Finally, in its devotion to nurturing the brain above all other organs in the body, the fetus sends its most richly oxygenated blood only to its brain and upper limbs. The blood that goes to the lower body is slightly darker and less rich in oxygen. This circulatory feat is facilitated by a hole between the left and right atria, which closes at birth.

Energetically the heart patients seemed still to be trying to direct their vitality primarily to their upper bodies and their brains, although their circulation was no longer supporting this effort. My theory is that, because of some prenatal trauma, cardiac patients never made the transition to a full-body energy flow. The later need to suppress their anger supported this pattern of focusing their energy in their upper bodies.

When I first started doing energy work I noticed that I seemed to operate—to initiate both thought and movement—from a rectangular space, the bottom border of which ran across my chest, just below my heart, and the top of which ran just above my head, encompassing the upper four chakras. I knew that this was stressful for me because I could feel a blocked, dead space in the center of my back and a constricted feeling in my chest that eased as I became more grounded. I also knew, once I started working with end-stage cardiac disease patients, that I would have been one of those patients if I hadn't done all the emotional, energetic, and nutritional work on myself that I had felt drawn to do. I often felt that it could have been my own chest being sawed open on the operating table, but for the healing in all these realms that I had experienced.

In the group my patients' hearts just seemed to want to lie down and resume a horizontal relationship to gravity. After all, isn't that what a heart attack is telling them? Isn't the heart saying, "Just let me lie down. I can't function in a vertical position any longer"?

Had they been able, I would have loved to have the LVAD patients do a very simple exercise of crawling on the floor, then pulling themselves up to standing, using a doorknob or a chair, as an infant finding his legs for the first time might do. My hunch was that this first movement toward independence, in the course of which the organs of the body shift from a horizontal to a vertical relationship to the floor and to gravity, would not be an easy or happy process for them. The first time I tried it myself, tremendous fear came up in me, and I realized that I had started walking before I was ready to because my mother had been so eager to have a precociously responsible child. I'd have liked to enable my patients to reexperience this transition and see how their hearts responded. This was impossible, both because of how sick and weakened they were, and because of the tubes coming out of the their bodies attached to huge pumping machines.

Group Healing

Instead, I tried to address their immediate discomforts by doing group healings, in which one patient would lie on the table in the surgical conference room in which we were working, and the rest would gather around, with hands on his body at various positions. This exercise turned out to be very successful in easing the pain that some of them felt from having a hunk of metal inside them.

Kenneth gamely volunteered to get on the table first. As I had done with Paul's leg, I showed him how to move the energy down his body from the place of painful throbbing under his rib cage, where I was lightly resting one hand. I felt a stab of emotional pain there in the back of my hand, but Kenneth resisted the idea that it involved some hurt from his past that needed to be addressed, and I didn't push it. As I moved the hand lower down, he said he felt the pain moving down as well, which completely surprised him. I told him to think of the pain as energy and to defuse it by expanding the field of that energy until it was as large as his whole body. He did so, and his breathing deepened as the pain swept away.

I had them do the color breathing I had learned at Kripalu, in which they imagined drawing each color of the rainbow, one by one, into a different chakra as they breathed. The quality of the energy in the room changed as each different color came into their spines, and I wondered if this phenomenon was related to the emotionally laden internal visioning we do when we dream. I also had them sense the energy field around each other's heads and around each other's hearts. One person would stand behind a seated partner and hold their hands about a foot away on either side of the head. "Now just bring your hands in very gently until you feel a slight pressure pushing out against them. Sort of a line you just don't want to cross. That's the beginning of the energy field." They were thrilled that they all could feel it, and their partners all felt heat or pressure as the hands started closing in. Some of them said it was very relaxing, and others tingly and exciting. Later they repeated the same exercise with the heart.

WHEN THE SURGEON SPEAKS

Bobby's was the second LVAD implant surgery I worked on. Like so many of the LVADs, he came in through the emergency room. I was in Dr. Oz's office when he got the call, and I actually went down to the ER to escort Bobby up to the fourth floor and tell him that I would be with him in the operating room. He was going in and out of consciousness but still managed to acknowledge this with gratitude.

What I noticed, once he was under and Dr. Oz had started to work, was how despairing he was. As I had come to expect, when the doctor first touched his heart, I got a feeling of childhood battles waged and lost in Bobby's chest. I also got a sense of acute pain in his left atrium and on the left side of his head. Above all, he seemed to just want to rest. I told him to endure the pain of hoping that things could be different, and I sang to him on bypass. Nothing seemed to help, and the heavy feeling remained.

"How's he doing, Julie?" Dr. Oz asked.

"Not very well, Mehmet," I said. "He's very depressed."

"He should be," Dr. Oz responded with exasperation. "He's about as close to death on the operating table as you can be and still be alive."

Suddenly I realized that Bobby was consciously resisting all the work being done to force him to choose life. He actually resented the surgeons' urgent need to have him survive the operation—a need that seemed to have nothing to do with him personally. I leaned over and whispered into his ear, "You don't have to live. It's up to you to decide. If you want to live, we're here to make that option available to you. But you don't owe us anything. You don't owe us your life." I felt him relax.

Dr. Oz remarked that he seemed to be doing better and asked me what I'd said to him.

I hesitated. "I felt that he was wandering back and forth between this world and the next," I said, "and that he wasn't sure he wanted to stay here. I also felt that he was really resenting the pressure you guys were putting on him to live. So I told him he didn't have to."

"*You did what!!?*" Mehmet said in horror. Then, before I could answer, he began yelling at the supposedly unconscious patient. "Mr. Fawcett," he screamed, "*You come back here.*" he screamed. "*I have important things to talk to you about!*" I felt Bobby brightening. Dr. Oz remarked that he was doing even better, although he was still bleeding severely. I felt that this stemmed from his need to show his father, whom Dr. Oz now represented, how badly he was hurt. I told Bobby to get the pain out of his blood and to give it to Dr. Oz, as he would have liked to give it to his father. I told him to put anger and aggressiveness in his blood instead. The bleeding gradually subsided.

After the operation I pointed out to Dr. Oz how important his angry caring and his personal connection was to Bobby. "He started to stabilize when I spoke to him, and told him it was his choice to live or die, but he really came back when you yelled at him and showed him how much you cared. Couldn't you do that with every surgery?" I asked.

"It's bad enough I have you in there, Julie," he said. "It would just be too embarrassing to do it on every case. The perfusionists and half of anesthesia are already laughing at me. You don't know the heat I'm taking for this."

TALKING TO THE ESTABLISHMENT

My final effort as a graduate student was a research paper, now six months overdue, on the introduction of alternative medicine into a large academic medical center, using Columbia as a model. My intention was to interview department heads, the president of the hospital, the deans of the nursing and medical schools, and possibly board members. I also planned to talk to some of the medical students who had been attending an elective survey course on alternative medicine that was being offered this year, in response to student demand, for the first time.

The paper would also cover what had been happening at the Rosenthal Center, my own experiences with the cardiothoracic surgery department, and a brief political history of the Office of Alternative Medicine at the National Institutes of Health (NIH). I included the last item because the mere formation of the office had clearly given alternative medicine a legitimacy without which none of this would be happening. I also felt it was important for people to realize the political realities surrounding alternative health care in this country—that it wasn't some overwhelming public demand that had brought the office into being but the experience with alternative medicine of one ex-congressman, whose close friend happened to chair the appropriations subcommittee for the NIH.

As I did my interviews, the political reality of what gets offered to patients became even more apparent. In terms of both utilization and information, the general public was clearly way ahead of those who had the most power and prestige in the medical world (the honchos at academic medical institutions, who set the tone for all medical practice). Most of the people I talked to were not even beginning to feel the grass roots of this movement tickling their feet. Until they did, I realized, little change in terms of allocation of resources would occur.

Among other things, the interviews gave me a much greater appreciation of the difficulty of Dr. Oz's position. Of the twenty-two people I talked to in positions of authority, half didn't even know that the Rosenthal Center existed, and only four knew the name of its director. Only one, the dean of the medical school, knew anything about its activities. No one knew the name of the director of the Office of Alternative Medicine at the NIH, or anything about what it was doing. Only three knew anything about what was happening with cardiac surgery patients, and one of them, the director of the Heart Failure Center, told me that it was "nothing but a hustle to attract more patients."

Among the people I interviewed, I was surprised to discover that only two had actually used alternative modalities themselves, and only three knew of friends and relatives who had. I asked each of them if they had some physical ailment or discomfort that Western medicine had been unable to adequately address, and most of them said yes. I then asked them whether, if an alternative therapy for that problem were made available to them gratis, they would avail themselves of it. To my complete surprise, all except the president of the hospital said no! This included five who said that they would like to see research done on alternative modalities in their specialties. I could only conclude that their spirit of scientific inquiry did not extend to their own persons.

William Speck, the president, was in fact one of the most open-minded of my interviewees. A pediatrician, he pointed out to me that doctors who deal with children are unique in the medical profession in that they tend to become advocates for their patients. He was sensitive to the despair and poverty in the streets that surround the hospital—a subject that no one else with whom I spoke addressed.

If he himself had a chronic, serious condition like cancer, he said, he would definitely seek out something in the alternative realm. For a brief moment I began to feel some hope for my future at the hospital. Then he told me how regrettable it was that the rising public interest in alternative medicine happened to coincide with such rough financial times for the institution, making it unlikely that unconventional therapies would be incorporated into the care it offers in the foreseeable future. Unless, he added, capitation, which makes it more profitable to keep patients out of hospital beds than in them, became the rule rather than the exception.

I was struck by both his candor and his warmth. Unfortunately, his assessment of economic priorities was echoed when I talked to Allen Hyman, chief of staff and medical director. "If we have to choose between a million-dollar imaging device, which will make us competitive in attracting patients, and a program of alternative medicine, which we have no indication will do that, we're going to spend the money on the machine," he told me.

Only after I left Hyman's office did I think of the calls and letters that poured into the Rosenthal Center every day, asking for advice about alternative modalities and wanting to know what Columbia Presbyterian was offering along these lines. David Eisenberg at Harvard had done a survey showing that one-third of all Americans were using alternative modalities and spending over $13 billion annually for them. I regretted not remembering and mentioning this point. But then, it would probably have made no difference. Somehow the enchantment with technology goes beyond economic realities, and the holy "bottom line" is invoked as much to support entrenched belief systems as to insure survival.

When I asked my interviewees about the most significant changes they had observed in medicine since the beginning of their practice, most cited the current economic climate. They seemed genuinely hurt, confused, and in some cases irate at the tightening of the public and private purse strings and at the "greed" of the HMOs. I didn't think it would be tactful to point out that the very generous remuneration most physicians and hospital administrators received was, perhaps, what gave the HMOs the notion that there was serious money to be made in medicine. Or that it was their own widespread habit of treating patients as if they were their diagnoses that initiated the "depersonalization" of medicine. They just never expected the depersonalization to extend to themselves. When the president of the hospital, discussing "belt tightening," told me that the unions would have to compromise, I knew he was not talking about the AMA.

One of the most interesting and lively people I interviewed was Bennett Stein, chief of neurosurgery and director of the Neurological Institute. He had heard about my work and invited me to tell him more about what I did in the OR. When I finished, he said with a twinkle in his eye, "Hearts are boring, Julie. Brains are fascinating. Why don't you come and work with us?"

ENERGY IN THE EMERGENCY ROOM

The director of the acute care section of the emergency medicine department had also invited me to come down and see if what I was doing might fit in in the emergency room. Following his invitation, I went down to the ER to observe for a day. I was particularly interested in doing so because this was the place where the hospital interacted the most dramatically and consistently with the people of the neighborhood, many of whom used the ER as their primary care physician. I spent a little time in the waiting room, furnished with rows of unwelcoming plastic chairs, whose nondecorator colors were made even less appealing by the glare of the fluorescent lights overhead. A television, tuned to a soap opera, blared in one corner, and people of every age sat or slumped in attitudes of pain, boredom, or despair. They were all nonwhite and mostly underdressed for the coldness of the day. Spanish appeared to be the language of choice.

I immediately had a vision of the healing that could take

place right there: an area could be cordoned off where people waiting to be seen by a physician could do energy work on each other, following instructions on a chart. Just touching the bottom of the foot and sending energy into the kidney meridian would have a calming and vitalizing effect. It might even get them talking to each other, rather than allowing their pain to isolate them.

I told the man conducting triage at the entrance to the acute care section the name of the person I was here to see, then followed him back into a crowded room, where people were lying on beds or sitting in chairs, separated by curtains. A small area was devoted to asthma patients who, as in all ghetto areas, are regular visitors to the ER. I recalled my earlier, unsuccessful attempts to get the director of an asthma research project at the hospital interested in some alternative approaches to what just about everyone acknowledges is an emotionally mediated condition but is never treated like one. Should I mention to the nurse the acupressure points that could stop an attack in a few seconds? Large Intestine 4, between the thumb and the index finger, and Conception Vessel 22, at the jugular arch of the throat. Remembering that I had been invited in only to observe, with some concern on the part of the ER director that I might actually try to touch a patient, I decided not to.

Instead, I started a conversation with a nurse who was caring for an alcoholic and psychotic patient with the DTs. I told her a little about what I'd been doing in cardiac surgery, and she volunteered that she had studied therapeutic touch, a form of energy healing brought into the nursing world by Dolores Krieger, a professor at the NYU School of Nursing. "Where did you study it?" I asked.

"Here at Presbyterian," she said. "A nurse offers a course a couple of times a year." This was the first I'd heard of it, and it sounded very promising. I wondered if any of the cardiac nurses would be willing to take it and do energy work on the patients.

"Do you use it a lot?" I asked, thinking how calming it would be for the psychiatric patients.

"I did at first," she said. "But then—I don't know. It looked so odd to everyone else. And there was so much pressure to just do my job, I felt self-conscious and just let it go." This story was particularly disheartening. What was the point of teaching the nurses how to do healing if there was no support for practicing it? I mentioned this to the director of the acute care section, who was relatively new to Columbia, and he told me that he would like to change the situation.

I also suggested since the hospital was designing a new emergency medicine facility, it should pay attention to noise control and try to use incandescent instead of fluorescent lighting. "It will make for much more relaxed patients," I told him. "And a more relaxed staff as well." He called me a few days later to say that the engineers had told him that things were too far along in the planning stage. It couldn't be done.

Chapter Seven

BRAIN CANCER
SURGERIES

It was some months before I took Bennett Stein up on his offer to come into his operating room and "work with brains." In
the interim he referred a couple of patients who had expressed
an interest in alternative medicine to me for pre-op and post-
op care. I was both fascinated with and captivated by Alexy, a
young man in his twenties, whose parents were Romanian im-
migrants. He was, I discovered, an accomplished artist who had
lost interest in his own work but was fascinated with the whole
subject of energy.

After one session he developed an almost obsessive belief in
my power to move energy in his body and heal him. His
mother, delighted that something had brought him out of his
despair, called me in tears and begged me to come in and do an
extra session with him before my next scheduled visit to the
hospital.

Alexy had had surgery for a tumor whose symptoms had
been debilitating him for years and that he was told would

eventually paralyze him. Since he'd had trouble regaining his strength and couldn't seem to keep any solid food down, he complained that Dr. Stein had deceived him and that the surgery had actually made him worse. I suggested that he start eating brown rice cream, and after a couple of energy sessions, he became capable of digesting it.

As I worked on him, focusing mostly on the head, spine, and legs, he told me about his life, which he considered to have been one of extreme dissolution. "I did drugs—wonderful visions. I went with women a lot. I was very cruel with them," he told me. It was quite believable. Even in his current emaciated state, he exuded a certain seductiveness and charm. "Now that I live at home," he said, "this is less possible. I didn't want to move back. My father had terrible rages and beat me very badly as a boy. He didn't understand. Of course, I forgave him."

But your body didn't, I thought to myself, knowing that the primary energy missing in his healing was the energy of his own anger. It was all held in his head, clouding his brilliance with obsession and paranoia. The penalty for standing up to his father must have been severe, I thought. He had had to contain his rage above the neck or at least in the spinal column. If it had come down into his body or out into his limbs, its presence would have led to action—to defending himself or running away, neither of which would have worked when he was a little boy and one-third the size of his oppressor.

I worked at his feet, trying to draw the energy down into his body, and insisted that he take at least a few steps around the room, which he succeeded in doing, before getting dizzy.

When I saw Dr. Stein again, he told me how much he appreciated the work I'd been doing with Alexy. "The psychiatrist had given up on him, Julie. We just didn't know what to do. But he's really responding to you." This news came as a surprise to me, because I considered my work with Alexy tantamount to a failure. I kept telling him that it was not my energy that was helping him, and I tried to get him to stay present during our sessions rather than zone out into an alpha state. What struck me was not how successful I was but how low the medical expectations were.

ENERGETIC BRAIN SURGERY

It was in December, almost a year after my first cardiac surgery, that I told Dr. Stein that I was ready to try working with him in the operating room. He suggested that I address the upcoming neurosurgical staff meeting, where most of the neurosurgeons and the two top residents would be present. A few minutes before the meeting was scheduled to start, he turned to me and announced, "I'm going to introduce you as a faith healer. Is that all right?"

I could see that all my careful explanations about the scientific principles behind what I'm doing had been for naught. Forget that the French physicist Louis de Broglie had discovered matter waves, which makes the concept that living tissue has a distinct vibratory energy pattern utterly plausible. Forget that proteins on the surface of a cell, which regulate much of its internal activity, respond to very low-level electromagnetic frequencies, as well as to chemical substances. Forget three thousand years of energy-based Chinese and Indian medicine, with just as high a cure rate as our own. To the chief of neurosurgery and the director of the Neurological Institute, it might all be a placebo effect.

"Dr. Stein," I said, as calmly as I possibly could, "my work does not depend on the belief of my patients. I have done healing successfully at a distance on people who didn't even know that I was working on them. The only faith that is necessary is my own. Would you please introduce me as an energy healer?" He seemed a bit disappointed but agreed.

In a few minutes his office was filled with men, most of them in white coats. Just before the meeting started, Evelyn, the departmental secretary, slipped in, only slightly relieving the gender imbalance in the room. The faces looked friendly, even interested, as Dr. Stein introduced me. "This is Julie Motz, who has been working over in cardiac surgery. She's, uh—she says she's an energy healer. I'm going to let her tell you about what she does. I thought it might be helpful for our patients."

Dr. Stein had asked me to be brief, so I gave a hurried description of my pre-, intra-, and postsurgical procedures. I stressed the fact that research had shown that the functioning of the auditory nerve is not diminished under anesthesia; only later did I realize that I was not likely to be standing at the patient's head, whispering into his ear, during brain surgery. I mentioned that with my methods patients go into and come out of surgery in a more relaxed way, and that they seem to relive old trauma when the body is opened and entered. I could sense a little discomfort in the room when I said this and even more when I talked about helping them process that trauma while the surgery was going on.

Dr. Stein remained friendly and relaxed and drew me out with questions. "How do you think this all works, Julie?" he asked.

"It's possible that when I touch someone with the intention of healing, I'm activating some as-yet-not-understood aspect of the nervous system or the endocrine system," I said, very much aware of the training and orientation of my audience. "These systems both may have energetic as well as chemical components to them." I was on fairly safe ground here, since no one knows just how either system does all the things they do. Just how the timing of nerve impulses and hormone production are managed is still a medical mystery.

"My own belief is that what we call consciousness is not localized in the brain. It exists in every cell, and possibly every molecule in the body. In fact, part of the definition of being a molecule in your body may be partaking of your consciousness." I was in much less secure territory here, but I pressed on.

"We know, for example, that cells are in constant communication with each other. They have to be, in order for billions of them to function in that incredibly efficient bureaucracy called the body. Furthermore, we know that these communications are happening faster than nerve impulses—they're not being directed by the brain. What I'm doing is simply tuning my brain's consciousness, and that of my patients, into those conversations, so we can have direct input."

Nothing in either biology or physics contradicts this idea—that is to say, the mechanism is scientifically plausible, even if not yet demonstrated. "We also know," I continued, "from the work of yogis, who can lower their heart rate and raise their body temperature at will—who can, in fact, sit naked comfortably in a foot of snow—that it is possible to have conscious control of what are normally considered unconscious bodily processes. We also know from experiments with biofeedback that anyone can be taught to do this to some degree. I believe that this is possible, even when a patient is anesthetized."

"Doesn't this depend on what the patient believes?" Dr. Stein asked. I was a little dismayed. I thought he and I had already gone over this territory, but he seemed strongly attached to this idea. "No," I said firmly. "A lot of my cardiac patients don't have a clue about what I'm doing when I start. They're just willing to try anything their surgeon says might help."

"Do any of you have any questions?" Dr. Stein asked, turning to the group. There was an awkward silence. Then one of the younger surgeons raised his hand.

"I do a lot of surgery for epilepsy," he said, "and it doesn't always work. Do you think you could help with that?"

"I'd certainly be willing to try," I said, wondering at my own arrogance.

"Thank you very much," Dr. Stein said, and I realized that my part of the show was over. As I closed the door behind me,

I longed to be a fly on the wall during the next part of the meeting. What did they make of all that? I wondered, suspecting that I'd gone too far.

The next day I called Evelyn, the departmental secretary, to try to get a reading on how it went. "About half of them were sort of interested," she said. "And the other half . . ."

" 'Not in my operating room,' right?"

"Right," she said.

Given this ambivalence, I was particularly pleased when Dr. Stein called me a couple of weeks later to tell me that he had a case for me. (Much later I learned that one of his colleagues had rushed to a phone immediately after the meeting to call a friend and say, "Stein has finally flipped his lid. He brought a faith healer to the staff meeting this morning.")

The patient was a woman from Delaware named Sandra with an arterial-venous malformation—the classic "bomb in the brain." Dr. Stein explained to me that this condition occurs when the capillaries that connect arteries and veins in some part of the brain are malformed. Arterial blood rushes across into a vein, which cannot withstand the pressure, and ruptures. The point of the surgery was to find the area of the bleeding, excise the blood vessels, and seal it off.

A few days before her surgery, I worked with Sandra, who was a mother in her thirties. What I felt more than anything else was a desire in her brain for rest. There was also a strange rushing feeling in the left front of her head, where the malformation had occurred. She was torn between worry and hope about the operation. She was also, in an almost endearing way, obsessed with keeping her bangs. I told her that although she would be unconscious when her head was prepared, I would convey her concern to Dr. Stein and to the barber and see that they were preserved. She seemed almost as grateful for this as for my energy work.

The neurosurgical operating room seemed even more packed with equipment than the cardiac rooms. Most striking was the apparatus that allowed the surgeons to look at the very delicate field of their work through binocular magnifying lenses and also on video screens strategically positioned around the operating table. Before this scope was wheeled into place, however, Sandra was eased up into a sitting position, and a drain to remove the spinal fluid that bathes the spinal cord and the brain was put in place at the bottom of her back. When this was done, she whimpered like a terrified child.

When she was lying down again, as the anesthesia was being administered, I worked intensely at her feet, not just touching them lightly as I usually do but massaging them vigorously, working on pressure points, trying to ground her and to soothe the sexual terror that seized her body as she went under. I told Dr. Stein about the bangs, and accordingly he had the barber shave off a patch of hair a little above the hairline on the left side. The head itself was held steady by a device that looked like something out of a medieval torture chamber, with pins that pierced the skin in a crown around the head. An incision was made just above this shaved area, and the skin was yanked down, revealing the naked skull.

As this was happening, I got a tangled and knotted feeling from Sandra's brain, and a sense that she was carrying a kind of craziness there for one of her parents, and that she shared it as a secret with her sister. I felt in her a deep sadness about it, which I told her psychically to let go of. As the scalp clips were put in place to hold back the skin, a feeling of longing for her father washed through her. As Dr. Stein began to drill into the skull, a light, euphoric sensation replaced the longing.

He removed a rectangle of bone, which would be wired back when the surgery was completed. The scope was wheeled into place, and I shifted my attention to one of the video screens, continuing to hold Sandra's feet, sometimes massaging them and sometimes just sensing the energy pouring through one or more of the six acupuncture meridians that terminate in the toes and the bottom of the foot. I noticed surges of sexual

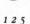

energy as Dr. Stein cauterized the feeder blood vessels at the surface of the brain and, as he went deeper, a strong charge on both the liver and the gallbladder meridians, which govern anger and pain. Throughout the surgery I got images of Sandra swimming.

No one had prepared me for the utter tedium of the surgery, which lasted for a little more than ten hours. Dr. Stein and a colleague worked rather like a wrestling tag team, spelling each other to stay fresh. Taking just one quick break to eat an apple, I was in the OR longer than anybody else.

When I visited Sandra in the neurosurgical ICU a few days later, she was comatose, and her husband looked desperate and frightened. The energy work had given me no clue about what was going on, but on an impulse, thinking about Alfred Tomatis's work, I bent over and started singing in a soft high voice very close to her ear, mostly just her name. After about five minutes she opened her eyes and looked at me with a clear, direct gaze.

Sandra seemed better for about a day, but staying conscious continued to be a struggle, and it soon became apparent that there was bleeding in the brain—it was either something new, or something that had been missed, for all the meticulous work of the surgery. I was not present for the re-op, but I saw her about a week afterward, and there was a terrible sorrow in her eyes. She started to weep as soon as I touched her.

She was not the kind of patient with whom I felt comfortable sharing the things I felt from her during the surgery. I sensed that they pointed to a path she would not want to travel, that she would prefer to think of what was happening to her as mysterious and unexplainable. I knew I had to honor this preference, but it made me uncomfortable, and I decided that in the future I would try to limit my work to people who, like myself, were willing to see illness as the bearer of information about oneself and one's personal or social history. As fascinating as the body in all its functions and dysfunctions might be, disease interested me primarily as a vehicle for personal transformation, for both patient and healer.

Sandra was in the hospital for two weeks after the second surgery, and I stopped in to see her again just before she was discharged. She was looking forward to going home with the intensity of a child anticipating Christmas, but I knew it would be to an uncertain life. A shadowy sorrow around her suggested that she knew it too. Seizures, which I believe are anger-related, are a very common aftereffect of these surgeries, and that threat was still hanging over her.

ANGER AND THE BRAIN

If it was people in search of personal transformation I was after, my next neurological case seemed to fit this requirement precisely. The patient, a former-corporate-lawyer-turned-part-time-clergyman-and-antiques-dealer, was referred to me by a colleague of Dr. Stein's who had heard me speak at the staff meeting. Less than two weeks after Sandra's surgery, he called me, saying he had a patient who was asking about alternative treatments for his brain tumor. Would I be willing to talk to him?

Walter was unlike any other patient I had met at Columbia so far. A very tall, attractive man with silvering blond hair and a boyish charm, he was extremely interested both in alternative therapies and in the possible psychological implications of his disease. I saw him and his wife together alone at first and then, on an impulse, invited them to come to a healing group I ran once a month for other healers.

He estimated from the onset of the symptoms, which included severe headaches, that his brain tumor had started about two years ago. "What was happening in your life then?" I asked.

"I put my parents in a nursing home and became responsible for taking care of them." He himself had already made the connection between the inception of the tumor's growth and his despair at that moment. He despaired that the conversation he had been awaiting for many years, the conversation in which he finally confronted his harsh and abusive father with the damage he had done, would now never take place. His father was too frail and sick.

One of my own theories, I told him, was that brain problems originate from asking the brain to perform a task that is really meant for the body. In his case, it was the task of holding anger, which is a natural energy of the body, specifically of the muscles. My hunch was that his entering the ministry represented an unsuccessful attempt to quell his angry thoughts.

Releasing some of this anger would help, I told him; his father's presence wasn't necessary. I had him stand facing a wall, with his feet about a shoulder-width apart, and instructed him to make fists, inhale, and say with every exhale, as forcefully as he could, "I'm angry."

Although this exercise is simple, it was not easy for Walter to do. Years of training, starting in childhood, had taught his musculature to relax instead of tense when he felt rage, so anger brought him no sense of strength. In fact, it put him into a state so close to parasympathetic shock (the hyperrelaxation of the autonomic nervous system) that even though he could intellectually acknowledge that he had things to be angry about, he literally didn't feel it. Instead he felt like fainting or falling asleep.

"I'm angry," Walter said obediently during the exercise, with all the enthusiasm and energy of someone reading a stock quote. I let him do this a couple of times, knowing that it would take time for the energy to build and for his body to hear and feel what he was saying.

"Breathe!" I said. "Breathing in brings the energy of fear and excitement into your body, the energy of perception, and a taking in of the outside world. You need the energy of fear to push the anger out." He took a deep breath and continued. "Say it angrily," I coached. "And if you don't think you feel it, pretend that you're an actor on stage, acting as if you're angry."

He seemed to connect with this, and his voice got a little louder and more forceful. Then, incongruously, he smiled. This often happens when people use this technique. It's a way of saying, "I don't really mean this."

"Don't take it back," I said. "Your life is not a joke, and the things that have hurt you, the things that make you angry, aren't funny. Smiling might have been a way to deflect someone's attention from your rage when you were a child, but it isn't protecting you and it's not working for you now. You have to take your own anger seriously, or nobody else will."

"I'm tired," Walter complained. "I can't go on."

"You've barely started," I said. "You're just beginning to connect. I know this is hard to believe, but there will come a point where this will be easy, and anger will just flow through your body like a power charge. Right now you're struggling with all the blocks your mother created in you, to keep you from ever confronting Daddy and feeling your own power." This seemed to hit home, and Walter took a deep breath and started again. His voice was now down below his throat coming from the middle of his chest. I put one hand on his solar plexus and the other on his back. "Keep moving your voice down into your body. Let it connect with your genitals. Aim the feeling down at the floor."

"I'm angry!" he yelled, actually raising his voice for the first time. I felt the energy moving down his spinal column in a rush.

"Good!" I said. "That's great." The next "I'm angry," predictably, was softer, almost pleading. "You don't have to beg," I said. "You don't need permission to do this. This is your feeling. Stick with it. Start pointing to yourself and emphasize the 'I.' "

"I'm angry!" Walter bellowed, and opened his eyes very wide, as if surprised by the sound of his own voice.

"Great! Keep it up!" I said, sensing that this was the beginning of the end of the tyranny of his father's anger, the memory of which had cowed him for so many years.

"I'm angry! I'm angry! I'm angry!" he said, all in one breath, then looked as if he would like to collapse.

"Just once on each exhale," I said. "Don't run ahead of the fear."

"*I'm angry!*" he said with a terrific blast.

"Again."

"*I'm angry! . . . I'm angry! . . . I'm angry!*" Walter yelled, taking a deep breath each time and filling the room with the energy of his voice. No trace of heaviness or fatigue remained now. His wife had been watching him, at first anxiously, then excitedly throughout this process. I told him to look at her. The moment their eyes met, the love came pouring out, and he began to cry.

"It's important for you to know that this has been witnessed, and witnessed lovingly," I said. "We know that your anger is a loving feeling—that it protects the most vulnerable part of yourself—and we love you for it." This was no exaggeration on my part. It would have been impossible to witness what Walter had risked and not feel a rush of warmth and affection for him. It wasn't just the knowledge that he had to battle back through decades of armoring and early threats of annihilation to get here—it was the feeling of safety and elation that his energy and courage created in the room.

A few days later Walter and his wife came to my friend Michelle's house for the healing group, which that day consisted of Michael, Michelle, Walter, and me. We talked about how the brain strains itself by trying to do the work of the body. "Anger and love, action and connection, are feelings of the body," I said. "Fear and pain, perception and understanding, are feelings of the brain." This piece of emotional information had come directly out of my encounter group experiences.

The more I was around other healers who did not share this

background in encounter groups, the more aware I became of how vital it was to the success of my work. It gave shape, form, and meaning to everything I did, allowing me to perceive patterns that were invisible to others. Most important, it meant that I didn't have to invoke angels, "guides," disembodied spirits, other-dimensional physics, or anything in the realm of the mystical to explain what I did.

Emotions are the energies that run both our lives and the universe. One day when I was discussing this with Sonja Gilligan, she playfully suggested that the basic forces in physics be renamed *fear, anger, pain,* and *love.*

"That would certainly get people used to the idea," I responded. With most of my patients, however, I did not discuss the larger implications of Sonja's theory. I just invoked the relevant pieces for those who gave evidence that they were open to a discussion of emotions.

Walter himself brought up the idea that his brain had been holding not only anger but love and sexuality as well. Michael put his hands on Walter's head, and Michelle knelt at his side and put her hands on his chest and his back. I sat at his feet, holding his big toes, strategically placing my index fingers at the inner corner of the nail, where the liver meridian, which carries the energy of anger, begins. My thumbs were on the outer corner of the nail—the entry point for the spleen meridian, which influences sexual energy.

Michael, who seemed the most tuned in to what was going on inside Walter, asked him what the energy felt like inside his head. "It's tight and twisted," Walter responded.

"I want you to go down to your groin and ask it what message it has for your brain," Michael instructed.

"It says, 'Unwind, let go!' " Walter said with a laugh.

"Do you think you could do that?" Michael asked.

"I could try."

"Try it now. Use our energy, the energy we're drawing into

your body, to make it safe." As Michael said this, I felt a rush of energy coming down the spleen meridians, along the outside of Walter's big toes, and a general relaxation in his whole body.

"That's it," Michael said encouragingly. "Just let it keep coming."

"I'm feeling a little dizzy," Walter said.

"Just breathe," I said, "and let yourself take in. This is new for you. You're used to being the caretaker, to taking care of everybody else's pain. Now it's your turn."

Walter began to cry, but the energy kept moving. I felt as if I'd floated up off the floor. Michael made a sound, like a cross between a very deep-toned bell and wind rushing through a cave. I had no idea how he did it, or where in his being it was coming from, but it moved through me with a delicious shiver, and I found myself chanting something back, higher and more vocal, as if it were coming from the back of my head. Michelle was now also making a sound somewhere between a low croon-ing and a howling, like a hound baying the moon. I wondered for a moment if Walter was thinking that we were all crazy and was longing to flee, but the feeling coming into my hands from his body was deep sorrow, moving into exultation, then back to sorrow, then into exultation again.

Suddenly, as if by some prearranged signal, we all stopped and took a deep breath. And all of us, including Walter and his wife, were smiling at each other. In fact, we were beaming. "Thank you," Walter said. "Thank you so much. I never could have imagined anything like this."

"Thank you," I said, with Michael and Michelle echoing my words. This was neither affectation nor mere politeness. Through his healing Walter had offered us all a way to connect to each other, and to all the loving energy in the universe. I sud-denly understood why surgeons tend to be such high-energy people: it was the healing they got from their patients. The ut-ter trust with which people go into surgery—the trust that is necessary when they give the care of their body and the responsibility for their life to someone they barely know—is a tremendous affirmation of love. Just by coming into the OR the patient, whether he acknowledges it or not, is expressing his love toward the surgeon. Allowing the surgeon to open and enter his body, while he, the patient, is utterly out of control, is an even deeper act of love. The only thing that comes vaguely close to it is sexual intercourse. How could a surgeon not be energized and, in fact, healed, by this love, as he touches and probes the body?

I did not share this insight with the surgeons I knew, but I dreamed of an operating room where this mutuality of healing was openly acknowledged. I talked about this with my friend Rory Block, a great blues singer with wonderful spiritual insights. "Going under anesthesia has to be a spiritual state, Julie," she said, "because there is no judgment."

I incorporated this idea into my preoperative sessions. "For the hours you are in surgery, you will not judge, and you will not be judged," I started saying, "and this state of nonjudgment is the highest spiritual state of all. It is a state in which great transformations can occur on many levels. I will be there to connect to that part of you seeking transformation as well as restoration, in every part of your being."

I longed to communicate this idea to anesthesiologists, to tell them that they were the ones bringing patients to this place. I mentioned it, almost casually, at the beginning of a few cases, hoping that at least one anesthesiologist would incorporate it into his "now we are going to sleep" patter, but it didn't take. Even mentioning spirit in an operating room made them a little nervous.

Still, the vision persisted. And as happens with everything in which I am denied, it grew. I pictured an operating room where surgery began with everyone in attendance thanking the patient for being there, and for bringing his love and trust into the room to create a healing space for us all. We would also thank him for giving meaning to our lives that day, because without him we would have no focus for our love and our knowledge. Finally each of us would commit to putting into the space of nonjudgment in which the surgery would occur whatever it was we needed to have healed at that time.

I thought about Dr. Oz's resident, pouring his bitterness and frustration into Donald's open chest during his bypass surgery, and wondered if my visionary surgery would have produced a different outcome. Treating the body as a machine is dangerous, and so is pretending that the people working on it are simply more competent and intelligent machines. No one can really leave his life or his personality outside the operating-room door. So-called "clinical detachment" is just a sham, and it seemed to me both unprofessional and unethical to endorse this charade.

Somehow—and I certainly don't know how—there has to be a space for dealing with people's feelings when they enter the OR. Not just the patient's feelings (which are usually ignored in any case) but everybody's feelings.

On the day of Walter's surgery, before the operation itself, the surgeon ordered a CT scan to determine the condition of the tumor. Lying in the scanner brought up memories of humiliation and helplessness for Walter, and the numbers four and seven came to me, possibly the ages associated with his memories. I felt the helplessness escalate into panic in his body and told him to send the fear, which was full of information, up into his brain. Looking at the scan, I felt rage coming off the screen and a sense of disgust, like a fear, sickening with inaction.

The tumor had almost doubled in size since the last scan; hearing this in the operating room, after the surgery had begun, brought great sorrow into Walter's brain. I told him to let himself feel all of it, then moved down to position myself at his feet, where I stayed for most of the operation. With my hands on his toes, I felt sorrow flowing through his liver meridian, which should have been carrying anger. I knew that this confusion of anger and pain in his body—this sorrowing when he needed to be raging—was at the heart of his energetic imbalance. When the head brace was pinned to his skull and he was put in a prone position on the table, a feeling of dull resignation came into his body, and I wondered if his father had beaten him from behind. My own impulse was to cradle him like a baby, and I held this image out to him energetically.

I decided to shift my position and sit with my head actually under the surgical drape, so I could place one hand at the base of his spine and one on the soles of his feet. A great rush of energy came down his spine as I did this.

The surgery was not nearly so long as the one I had done with Dr. Stein, but it also went very slowly, compared with the high-action, high-drama pace of a cardiac operation. The surgeon took tiny pieces out of the brain, which seemed to be experiencing some sorrow at the loss. When he had enough to biopsy, the scrub nurse handed it off to the circulating nurse, holding it between oversize tweezers called, descriptively, pickups and dropping it into a plastic cup, which the circulating nurse then labeled for the pathologist. I left my position at Walter's side and went over to put my hands around the container to sense the energy of the tumor. I got a feeling of compacted, vibrating rage.

To my surprise, as I was holding the specimen, the surgeon looked up from his work and asked me what I was doing. "I'm trying to get a feeling of its energy," I said.

"What did you feel?"

"Compacted rage," I answered.

"Is that what you always get?"

"Not with all tissue, but with malignant tissue, yes."

A few minutes later a strange drowsiness came over me, very similar to what I had experienced in the operating room with Barbara. I checked in with Walter, who seemed to be present, and then I noticed that the anesthesiologist was nodding on his stool, on the verge of sleep. The energy level in the room had

Hands
of
Life

dropped, and the key to this was what was going on with the surgeon. My mentioning the anger in the tumor tissue seemed to have put him into a state of withdrawal, deep inside himself.

I felt it would be indecorous to point this out to him; he could obviously continue to operate with skill and efficiency even in this low-energy state. I also thought it would be unwise to go over and shake the anesthesiologist, who didn't have very much to do during this part of the surgery in any case. Instead, I started a conversation with the surgeon, which seemed to raise the energy level again. "What will you recommend after the surgery?" I asked.

"Radiation," he said. "There's no way we can be sure of getting it all now."

"Doesn't that damage normal brain cells as well?" I turned to ask the anesthesiologist, who was now sitting up straight and alert, in a low voice.

"Yes, but those effects are noticeable only after a few years. With a fast-growing glial blastoma, they don't expect the patient to last that long. At some other hospitals they just do nothing, but the policy here is always to radiate."

I was horrified and suddenly in a panic. When Mike and Sonja's son, Patrick, was autopsied, I remembered, the radiation appeared to have done most of the destruction in his brain, not the tumor. What would I tell Walter about all this? And how much of this was privy information, not meant to be communicated to the patient?

I saw Walter in the neurosurgical ICU after the surgery. His son was also there, and I made a critical and, as it turned out, tactically disastrous decision to tell him what I had learned. "How did it go?" Walter asked.

"It's a very fast-growing glial blastoma," I said, "which means they don't expect you to live longer than a year." His son glowered at me. "They're going to recommend radiation," I continued, "which will probably damage normal tissue as well."

I knew that Walter had already made plans to see a macrobiotic counselor and to pursue other alternative treatments, and I hoped my information would persuade him to stick to that course. "We won't tell Mom, will we?" said his son. Having met Walter's wife, I knew that she would want to know, would want to share everything with him. It was his own pain and terror at the thought of losing his father that Walter's son was trying to keep in check.

When I came back a few days later to do a postoperative session, Walter and his wife were meditating in silence in his room. I waited respectfully at the door until they were finished, then stepped inside, feeling distinctly like an unwelcome intruder. I had been agonizing over what I had told Walter. *Couldn't you have kept your mouth shut, Julie?* I chided myself. *Couldn't you have let the surgeon give them the news?* But my panic about Walter's being whisked from surgery into radiation had been too great.

I started to apologize, telling Walter how driven I was by my own terror, but he cut me off. "I felt as if you were giving me a death sentence," he said. "That's not what I needed to hear." I didn't bother to defend myself or lay out my reasons. I understood his bitterness. And why not kill the messenger? It's a time-honored tradition. His wife, trying to smooth things over, told me that his recovery from the surgery had been remarkably swift, and everyone had commented on it. I left without doing the postoperative session, feeling that anything I could offer at that time would be unwelcome. Walter told me that his son had been investigating a new treatment, some kind of combination of chemotherapy and radiation that they were trying out down at NYU, and that he would probably transfer himself down there.

In spite of Walter's quick recovery, I left feeling discouraged and useless. "He asked you how it went, Julie," my cousin Michael reminded me. "He said he wanted to know. You did what was ethically correct, and what felt right to you at the time." It helped a little, but I realized with some pain how invested I was in having my patients think that I'm wonderful, at all times and in every way. I couldn't bear to think I'd disappointed them. I needed their love much more than they need my healing, I thought.

Chapter Eight

⌒〜⌒

BREAST CANCER
SURGERIES

Several months before I started working in neurosurgery, I was thinking about ways to branch out and work with other surgeons in other areas. John Matthews, who had been rotating through surgical training as part of the third-year curriculum, reported back to me about his experiences in other operating rooms. He was particularly taken with the work of Alison Estabrook, chief of the Breast Service, who took a lot of time explaining to students what she was doing and why. I had heard promising things about Freya Schnabel, Dr. Estabrook's partner, from the director of the Rosenthal Center, who felt that her deep religious commitment (she is an Orthodox Jew) made her more open than doctors usually are to ideas about spirituality and healing.

A friend of mine was on the board of a small family foundation that funds alternative cancer therapies. I had been talking to him about my work with cardiac patients and asked him if there was a chance that the Symington Foundation would give me a grant to do similar work with breast cancer patients. He seemed excited about the idea, and so I called Dr. Estabrook and Dr. Schnabel and set up a meeting.

They were both warm and enthusiastic. "We're in favor of anything—anything—that could help our patients," Freya Schnabel told me. "I think a number of them would be open to this." I suggested that I observe a surgery first, and then do a surgery with one of them, before applying for the grant, just so I could feel confident that the work really would be significant and could write convincingly to the foundation to that effect.

A few days later I watched most of an excisional biopsy (where a small lump is taken out and examined for malignancy) that Dr. Estabrook performed on a woman in her fifties. The calmness and quiet in the room were a distinct contrast to the clamor and noise and the sense of imminent emergency in the cardiac rooms. By accident or by design, all those present were women. When I tuned in to the patient, I felt sorrow draining off the operating table onto the floor from the place where the breast lump was removed, and I decided then and there that this was an area in which I wanted to work and in which major healing could be done.

As the patient came out of the anesthesia, Dr. Estabrook's physician's assistant, Mary Beth, was bending over her. "Thank you," she said to Mary Beth, "thank you so much. And thank you," she said, tilting her head back to look at the anesthesiologist. A feeling of warmth, love, and acceptance suffused the room, and a feeling of being nurtured. Dr. Schnabel had told me that the wonderful thing about being a breast cancer surgeon is that you follow your patients for the rest of their lives. How different this seemed from the world of cardiac surgery.

A Burden Removed

A few weeks later I got a call from Vanessa. She told me that soon after being diagnosed with breast cancer, she had seen an article in *The New York Times Sunday Magazine* describing my work. She was scheduled to have surgery with Dr. Estabrook and wanted to know if I would work with her.

I liked Vanessa the moment I saw her in Dr. Estabrook's waiting room. Her strength and calmness were very appealing, although she told me that she was very nervous about the surgery. She had been trying to follow a low-calorie vegetarian diet but without much success. I suggested that she eat as close to a macrobiotic model as possible and cut out dairy, which Chinese medicine considers a contributory factor in diseases involving the breasts and reproductive system.

I did a standard energy chelation on her but spent extra time at her solar plexus, the location of the third chakra, which governs, among other things, immediate family relationships. I felt a barrier there that I sensed connected to her mother. It seemed to be keeping the energy from flowing smoothly down to her pelvic area. I mentioned this to her, suggesting that this block might be what was keeping her from taking off weight. She said that her mother hadn't had much time for her; I felt a wrenching in her gut as she said this, then a relaxation.

On the day of the surgery I met Vanessa in the holding area outside the operating room. As we entered the OR, I saw that it had tiled walls in mushroom gray, which felt quiet and soothing. The anesthesiologist worked to put in the IV lines, and I felt panic and sorrow in Vanessa's body. The feelings persisted even after she was unconscious, mostly in the area of her solar plexus. As I had felt so often before with surgical patients, her sense of herself as a helpless child seemed to overwhelm her.

The surgery was a modified radical mastectomy, which meant that Vanessa's entire right breast would be removed and a sampling of lymph nodes taken for biopsy from under her arm. She seemed, in our preoperative session, to have no regrets about losing the breast, which was an unusual attitude for breast cancer patients. "A least it's not an arm," she told me.

I stood in my usual position, with my hands on Vanessa's temples, as Dr. Estabrook made a wedge-shaped incision in the skin of the breast, as if she were cutting a piece of pie. Then, using an electric cauterizer, she carefully worked her way around the breast in a circle, cutting away as much tissue as she could, exposing muscle below and skin above, thoughtfully pointing out anatomical markers to me as she did so. As she began to free the tissue over the pectoralis major, the muscle under the outer edge of the breast, I felt rage welling up in the area. I leaned over and told Vanessa to send the anger down into her leg; after I felt it moving there, I told her to let it spread over to the left side of her body. As she did so, a lightness took over her being. "You don't have to hold your anger in check, keeping it tightly in one place," I told her. "You can allow your whole body to experience it as forward-moving energy."

Dr. Estabrook began removing lymph nodes, being careful to leave the nerves under the arm intact. I sensed sorrow as the body let go of them, then of lightness and love. I got an image of Vanessa as a happy child, skipping down a treelined street. Soon afterward the breast was finally removed, and I felt the weight of a tremendous burden being lifted from Vanessa's body, although the breast itself was quite small. An image of an older woman, who I knew instinctively was Vanessa's mother, came to me. I knew then that it was her mother's feeling of being burdened by this child that Vanessa had been holding in her own breast all these years and that was now being released.

I leaned over and said softly into Vanessa's ear, "You were a delightful child, but your mother experienced you as a burden. You have held her feeling about you in your own breast for all these years. With your breast leaving your body, you can let go of that feeling at last."

By the time we got to the recovery room, Vanessa was fully

conscious and wanted to know everything I experienced with her during the surgery. I was a little hesitant to talk about her mother, and so I told her rather cautiously that I felt a great burden being lifted from her body when the breast was removed.

"What was it?" she asked.

"I felt that you were an utterly delightful child, full of love and energy. In fact, I got a wonderful image of you skipping down the street," I said. "But I also felt that in spite of this, your mother experienced you as a burden and was very bitter about it."

"She did, and she was," Vanessa said.

"I told you that when the breast left your body, this sense of having been a burden to her would be removed."

"I so hope that it was!" she said excitedly.

I saw Vanessa the next day for a post-op session, just before she was discharged, and we focused energy on the site of the surgery and her right arm. Three weeks later I got a wonderful letter from her, telling me that she was still talking to her body and using the imagery we worked with and that she was able to get by without using any pain medication after the surgery. She concluded by writing that she was following my dietary suggestions and her weight was going down. "I expect to be healthy and lean—but not mean!" she wrote. I smiled to myself, thinking of the little girl skipping down a treelined street.

Encouraged by these two experiences, I decided to go ahead and apply for a grant from the Symington Foundation to do healing work with women undergoing surgery for breast cancer. I received the grant in December 1995, just about a year after I first stepped into a cardiac operating room and around the time I started my work in neurosurgery.

Chemotherapy and Radiation

In spite of the deceptive quietness and relative simplicity of breast cancer surgery, where the time under anesthesia could be as short as an hour, no major body cavity was opened, and relatively little blood was generally lost, most breast cancer patients felt a hysteria about the disease itself, for which my experience with Vanessa did little to prepare me. I was much less aware of entering the world of hearts, when I entered cardiac surgery, than I was of entering the world of breasts, with all their significance in our society, as I began to work with women suffering from this disease.

Although I'd had a couple of cancer patients in private practice, cancer had never been a primary focus of my work. Now the whole arena of oncology, with its brutal and much too rarely successful solutions, was suddenly put before me. Working as I was squarely within the conventional medical system, I wondered what I would tell patients who asked me what to do about a doctor's recommendation that surgery be followed by chemotherapy and/or radiation.

This was never an issue with heart patients. With the singular exception of George, who courageously reduced his own medication when he, and not his doctors, figured out that it was ruining his kidneys, they were not in the habit of asking me about alternatives to the drugs prescribed for them after surgery. Nor, for the most part, were those drugs quite as likely to kill or debilitate them as their disease was. Of course, I would have liked to see them try changing their diets and dealing with their emotional issues instead of popping antihypertensive pills. I would have liked to see dandelion tea used after surgery as a diuretic instead of lasix. I would even have liked to see transplant patients using imagery to help keep the body from rejecting new tissue, instead of large doses of heavy-duty immunosuppressant agents like cyclosporin, or at least some experiments done using imagery and reduced dosages.

But these were my own ideas, and easy ones to keep to myself. Cardiac patients didn't agonize, as some cancer patients did, about whether they were uselessly sacrificing quality of life for no real guarantee of extended life. The majority of cancer patients with whom I worked went unquestioningly from the operating room to the chemotherapy drip or the radiation chamber. But just enough of them agonized about their choices to make me wonder just what I was doing there, what I should be doing there, and how much good I could do them if I didn't challenge some of the basic premises of their treatment.

The first problem, to my surprise, was actually getting the cases. I had given a number of the Columbia surgeons who routinely did breast cancer surgery stacks of material about my work and the Symington grant, but despite their smiles and assurances, they did not hand the material out to their patients on a regular basis. This astonished me, primarily because I still didn't quite register the degree of culture shock that my very presence in the hospital represented for most of its staff. My work with patients both in and out of the operating room seemed so natural and logical to me that it never occurred to me that it should gain anything less than total acceptance by the doctors—at least on the level of offering it to their patients when it had no medical downside and would cost them nothing.

But such acceptance was not to be—not even with Dr. Estabrook and Dr. Schnabel, who, I discovered, waited for a patient to mention some kind of interest in alternative medicine before bringing up the subject of having a healer in the operating room. How likely was a patient to bring up the subject, I wondered, when David Eisenberg's survey on the public's use of alternative therapies had revealed that most people using them were afraid to say so to their doctors?

I talked about this problem with Devita Deutsch, a dynamic woman with an energetic manner and sparkling, explosive eyes, who had started a breast cancer support group at Columbia. "I can't even get doctors to refer women to the group, Julie!" she told me, her voice full of concern and frustration. "Even with the published evidence that it extends lives." Devita was busy trying to convince her insurance carrier, which willingly paid for expensive reconstructive surgery after breasts had been removed, that they should be willing to pay for more than just one prosthesis, or set of prostheses, for women who didn't want to have their breasts reconstructed.

"They wear out. The average woman will probably need three in her lifetime, at a cost of a few hundred dollars—compared to thousands for the surgery. But men seem to think that women should want to have their breasts rebuilt—I guess because of what breasts mean to men. That, they're willing to pay for." Devita, an engine of intelligence, first-class rhetoric, righteous indignation, and persistence would eventually win her battle. But she had no suggestions for me about how to loosen up the surgeons.

With the clock on the grant ticking and no cases coming in, I despaired of Columbia and called Steve Horowitz, the chief of cardiology down at Beth Israel Medical Center in lower Manhattan. I had met Steve the previous spring, when I was despairing of finding a cardiologist at Columbia whom I could interest in some of my theories about early causes of heart disease. I asked him if I could send him some material describing my work with cardiac patients, then come see him. He agreed, and the meeting turned into a minidemonstration of energy healing, to which he was receptive. The politics of the situation at Beth Israel did not allow for introducing anything quite so far out to the patients yet, but we agreed to think about some way of working together. So almost a year later, when I called him looking for breast cancer surgeons to work with, he immediately suggested a friend of his, Shana Morris.

A few days later I got her on the phone, and she sounded warm, friendly, and—like Dr. Estabrook and Dr. Schnabel—interested in anything that might help her patients. I sent some material to her office, and about a week later her assistant called to tell me that a patient named Tracy who was scheduled for surgery wanted to work with me.

When I called Tracy, she told me that she had read about my work and was very excited about what I was doing. The path that had brought her to have this particular surgery with this particular surgeon at this particular time was so circuitous and unique that, she told me later, she thought the whole purpose of it may have been to bring us together.

The Crisis in Nurturing

Tracy was the first surgical patient I saw who had actively pursued some kind of alternative healing before seeing me and who firmly believed that, given time, it would work. She was also, however, feeling a great deal of pressure from her family and friends to have the surgery, as well as pressure from the surgeon. So she agreed, in spite of the fact that even without the benefits of surgery, chemotherapy, and radiation, she had already considerably reduced the size of the two lumps in her right breast.

An attractive woman in her early thirties, Tracy had bright red, curly hair and an athletic confidence to her body. Once she sat down on the couch in my living room, her story came exploding out of her, and she often raced over her feelings in an effort to make certain she told everything that had happened to her. Part of my work was simply slowing her down and pointing out sadness, rage, or fear as it welled up through the torrent of words.

Her disillusionment with the medical profession, in whose grasp she now found herself, was profound. Her position was very much like that of a child, having to go along with her parents' decisions about her well-being even though she no longer really trusted them. There was simply no one else big enough, powerful enough, socially validated enough to take over that sacred office, and when she dared to challenge them on the basis of her own instincts and experience, they knew exactly what buttons to push to frighten her back into compliance—mostly through implying that they had so much more information than she could possibly have. The words "for your own good" may form the single most suspect and dangerous phrase in the language.

The lumps in her breast, she told me, first showed up on a mammogram and then on a sonogram in the spring of 1994. She was told that they were just cysts and that they would go away. Instead they grew. A year later they were palpable through several layers of clothing, and a biopsy done at the end of March 1995 revealed that both were cancerous. The recommendation was for a modified radical mastectomy, probably followed by chemotherapy. A second opinion from another surgeon, who was not on her health plan, confirmed this plan.

This surgeon recommended Shana Morris, who, once more, confirmed the diagnosis, and surgery was scheduled for May 8. "I had no interest in doing anything else at that point," Tracy told me. "I didn't know a thing about alternatives and was all set to go ahead with the standard treatment. Then, about two and a half weeks before the operation was supposed to take place, I was in the dressing room at gymnastics class, telling the other students about the surgery, when one of them said, 'You should really see Karen.' At that point I didn't know what Karen did. All I knew was that she was a gymnast, and that she did—well, something that was supposed to help with injuries. In fact, I had been thinking about going to see her for a pain and a weakness in my Achilles tendon.

" 'Get serious,' I said. 'This is breast cancer. What could she possibly do for me?' Still, this woman was very insistent, so I decided I had nothing to lose. I called Karen, who explained something to me (which I barely understood) about jin shin jitsu."

Jin shin jitsu is a form of acupressure, using a limited number of points and always activating at least two at the same time, to create an energy flow. I don't agree with all its principles and feel it is weakest in its formulaic attempts to address emotional issues, but on the level of specific remedies for physical situations, I have been impressed with its power.

"I asked Karen what would happen if I came to see her," Tracy said, "and she told me that the lumps would go away. Of course I didn't believe her. I thought it was amusing that she even proposed such a thing. But feeling, as I said, that I had nothing to lose, since I was about to get my breast cut off in any case, I started seeing her anyway. I saw her twice on the following day, and on the day after that I went to see her teacher, Lillian Monroe. By the end of that third session there was a noticeable change in the size of both lumps. I was astonished.

"I kept seeing Karen once or twice a day, and the lumps continued to shrink and soften, although not so drastically as in that one session with Lillian. She also suggested that I work on myself, which you can do with jin shin, but I was too intimidated and insecure. I didn't think that I could really be effective doing it.

"I had to see Dr. Morris a few days before the surgery to have her draw on my chest just where the incision would be. The plastic surgeon who was to do the reconstruction had asked me to do this, then show it to him so he could be certain that he could work with it. By then I was impressed enough with the jin shin results that I wanted to give it a fair shot, so I asked Dr. Morris what would happen if I postponed the surgery for six weeks. She wasn't happy with the question, but since she couldn't give me a clear answer about any increased risk, I decided to postpone it from May 8 to June 19.

"The lumps continued to change texture and decrease in size, as if they were disintegrating. In fact, there was now a depression where one of them had been protruding from my breast. I gained a little courage and started working on myself as well. By the end of six weeks, one lump couldn't be felt at all, and the other was much smaller, less dense, and not so close to the skin. The Friday before the Monday of the surgery, I went to see Dr. Morris expecting she would do handsprings because one lump was virtually gone—just a raised circle in the skin, surrounding the area where it had been. Instead, she said, 'You're still coming in on Monday, aren't you?' I couldn't believe that was all she had to say!

" 'But one lump is gone!' " I said.

" 'But the other one is still there,' she countered. I didn't know what to say. She was ignoring what was happening in my body. I asked her if any other woman's lumps had ever changed as much as mine had, and she said no. I don't remember much else about the visit, because I was too stunned. Her point was that the cancer could still be there and could be spreading. I know that she was very scared, and that she felt that she was protecting both herself and me. Here I was, a young woman, only thirty-two, who had been completely healthy her whole life except for this. But still she ignored what was happening in my body. And she did what she was supposed to do—she scared me again.

"I called Lillian and asked her, 'What if it's spreading?' She assured me that I was doing fine and that it couldn't be spreading. Still, I left the hospital feeling very depressed and worried. Dr. Morris called my husband at work to get him to use his influence with me to have the surgery, but I canceled it anyway. I got some support from friends who believed in both my intelligence and my integrity—who knew that I was neither crazy nor so vain about my body that I couldn't bear to give up a breast. Who also trusted my sense that Karen and Lillian were legitimate in their healing practice, not just after my money, but genuinely concerned with the health and well-being of my body, mind, and soul."

Tracy's remark made me think about the general accusation that many alternative practitioners are concerned only with separating gullible people from their money—as if every test, procedure, and examination performed by a physician or a medical technician were of direct proven benefit to the patient and were never ordered or executed with any pecuniary motive. Why do some people assume that licensure is a guarantee of morality?

"That summer I took a seminar in jin shin jitsu. It was a wonderful experience. I continued seeing Karen once or twice a week and continued to work on myself. The lump and the raised circle where the other lump used to be continued to get smaller. In addition, my Achilles tendon no longer hurt; my hands and feet, which had always been cold, were now warm; my back wasn't stiff when I got up in the morning; and everyone, including my mother"—not, as I would subsequently learn from Tracy, a woman given to excessive praise—"said I looked younger and healthier.

"I hadn't been back to see Dr. Morris because she had told me at the end of my last visit that even if both lumps were to disappear completely, she would still want to take off the breast. 'What if I got a mammogram and a sonogram?' I asked. 'Mammograms in women your age are inconclusive,' she replied. I found this absurd.

"Even so, by the end of December there was still a raised circle of skin where one lump had been and something left of the other one. I decided this was taking too long, and that I would have a lumpectomy to get rid of them. I thought about finding another surgeon, but a woman I met through a breast cancer support organization had been a patient of Dr. Morris's and assured me that she would work with me and do whatever I wanted, even if she didn't approve of it. So I went back to Dr. Morris for a lumpectomy, without any lymph node dissection. I didn't let her take out the nodes because I understood that removing them would be just for diagnostic purposes, and I didn't want her to damage my arm just for that. I knew, no matter what the diagnosis, that I wasn't going to go ahead with chemo, which was what she would have recommended if there were enough positive nodes.

"On February 5 she took out what was left of both lumps, some tissue between the lumps, and a nodule she discovered behind my nipple. On February 13 I went for a post-op visit, and Dr. Morris told me that the cancer had gotten worse. Did this mean that the nodule and the space between the lumps were places it had spread to, where it hadn't been before? She couldn't tell me because nobody had checked there before. Although she had taken everything cancerous that she had seen, she insisted on a mastectomy because, as she said, 'It might still be there.' She said she wouldn't let me leave her office without making an appointment for the surgery.

"I was devastated. I felt beaten. I was surprised by the presence of the cancer in the two new places. And I was not expecting to have a mastectomy. Dr. Morris also said that she had to take out lymph nodes for 'local control' of the cancer, because the pathology report said that there were tumor emboli in my lymph vessels. So I agreed to have a modified radical mastectomy on February 26. But I kept thinking, 'There has to be something else that's going to happen. I couldn't possibly just be back where I started from, facing the same thing I was facing a year ago, a modified radical followed by chemotherapy. Something else has to be going on. I've learned too much and I've come too far.' "

A week before the surgery, Tracy got a call from Shana Morris's assistant, asking if it would be all right for me to be in the operating room with her. As Tracy told me, "I'd seen an article about you the summer before. I thought, 'Oh, my God, this would be phenomenal.' I told the assistant yes, and when I got off the phone, I was ecstatic. I knew then that this was why I was supposed to get the surgery done now—to meet you and to work with you. I was flying. You called me later, and we talked for a while. It was too late then for me to call a lot of other people, but I called a few and I told them, 'You can't believe this. This is going to be wonderful.' "

I was a little overwhelmed, since this was the strongest endorsement I'd ever had from someone who had never worked with me. It emboldened me to deal with Tracy sooner and more directly on an emotional level than I usually did with surgical patients. It came out, as we spoke, that her marriage was in serious trouble and that she felt isolated, unsupported, and alone. She anticipated that when the surgery was over, her husband would not even want to look at, let alone touch, the scarred side of her chest. This sense of isolation seemed to go way back, and from this very confident young woman, a portrait of a lonely and unvalued child emerged.

My heart ached for her, as it would over and over again for my breast cancer patients. Eventually I came to see the disease itself as a ghastly expression of the crisis around nurturing that the whole society is experiencing: a tortured longing to be loved.

In spite of all the lip service paid to "family values," we continue to underreward nurturing activities like parenting, teaching, and nursing. Traditionally men went into medicine, presumably from some desire to take care of their fellow, suffering human beings—to nurture them. And yet the medical education and training system we have created brutally suppresses and ignores the value of compassion as a healing tool. And so physicians come out officially stamped as "healers," with the guarantee that they will never be required to risk any of the feelings that go along with that title. How ironic; how typical of our society.

On the day Tracy came to my house for her preoperative session, the power had gone out. By the time we finished talking, it was dark, and I led her upstairs by candlelight to lie down on my massage table and experience what would happen to her in surgery on the next day. I put my hands on the tops of her feet and told her to allow herself to feel very light, as if her body were made out of clouds and the table were made out of clouds—as if she were actually floating down through the table.

"Now imagine that you're lying on a gurney, being wheeled

very gently and lovingly through the hospital corridors, into surgery."

"But I hate hospitals," Tracy said. "They do terrible things to people there. That's where people get sick and die. That's where they're going to cut off my breast."

"Everyone who works there, consciously or unconsciously, wants to be involved with healing. From the president of the hospital down to the janitor, they're all there because they want to help people, to be part of the healing process. Just remember their love and concern, and let it come into your body." I felt her breathing in and relaxing into this idea.

I once had a fight with someone up at Columbia who was designing a protocol for hypnosis for surgical patients. "Have them affirm that the anesthesiologist is filled with love, and that this love flows into them, along with the chemicals in the IV," I said.

"Are you crazy, Julie? You know how indifferent those guys can be."

"Some of them are and some of them aren't. But if the patient affirms that they are loving, it makes it safer and more possible for them to risk that feeling with him," I insisted. I did not win the battle.

"I want you to see yourself in the holding space outside the operating room," I continued with Tracy. "The anesthesiologist is putting in the needles."

Tracy flinched. "I hate needles."

"Pain is not punishment," I told her, since patients who were hit as children always associate the two. "Feel him putting the needle in so gently that it is like being massaged on the inside of your vein. Allow the needle to actually relax the vein, and realize that this is your channel of connection and communication to the outside world." Again I felt her relax.

"As you go under, I want you to split your consciousness. Send most of yourself to someplace warm and beautiful, where you really want to be, and leave just enough in the operating room to help Dr. Morris with the surgery."

How the hell do I do that? Tracy wondered.

Then, although I hadn't heard her thought, I said, "You know that you can do this because this is exactly what happens when you are reading a book. You're caught up in the story, but you still know that it's snowing outside."

I then told Tracy to relax her throat as the anesthesiologist puts in the breathing tube. "What do you mean, they're going to put a tube down my throat?" she said in a mild panic. "Nobody told me about that!"

"It's standard procedure," I said, "so that you can breathe, even though the muscles of your diaphragm will be relaxed. Just relax your trachea and let the tube come in."

"How do I do that?" she asked. "How do I relax it?"

"Just think about it," I said.

She did—and felt her entire throat and the upper part of her chest relax completely. "I couldn't believe it," she told me later.

"Now feel them painting your skin with betadine, to sterilize the area. And just before Dr. Morris makes the incision, just before she comes into your body with complete wisdom and complete love, I want you to send the blood away from the site of the surgery, pooling it in your extremities, to cut down on the bleeding."

"I have no clue how to send the blood to my extremities," Tracy said.

We know that words have the power to move blood around in our body, I explained, because when someone says something that embarrasses us, we blush.

Tracy decided to give it a try, and suddenly she felt as if her hands and feet were so heavy with blood that she could barely move them.

I described the incision with the scalpel, and the rest of the

Hands
of
Life

cutting with the Bovie. As the breast was leaving her body, I told her to thank it for all the pleasure it had given her and all the nurturing it had done. Although the breast was leaving, I said, that nurturing and loving energy would remain in her chest, and people would feel it emanating from her just as strongly. I also told her to thank the breast for giving up its life so that she could go on living, and living more securely.

Then I told her to let go of the lymph nodes and to allow to come into consciousness whatever memory they had been holding. I told her to feel the drainage tubes coming into her body, also to help her heal. Finally I told her to feel Dr. Morris stitching her up again with great care and concern, as flesh gratefully came together with flesh, and skin with skin.

Tracy later described her experience on the table that night as "the most mind-blowing of my life. Jin shin was very subtle," she told me. "I always felt very relaxed during a session. But with you, the moment I lay down, I felt as if there were an electric current running from head to toe."

After the surgical prep, I did a little work at her head. She experienced the energy there as being so strong that she asked me if we could stop soon—she didn't think she could take much more of it. It took her a while just to come back to the reality of the room and to open her eyes, and she needed my help in sitting up.

When she sat up, her hands were stiff and immovable, like a palsied person's in spasm. "I guess you could drive home like that," I said, and she laughed, releasing the tension in them just a little. But I was stumped about just how to relax them.

I stood her in front of a mirror and had her look at her hands. This released a little more of their tension, but she still couldn't move them. "Sit on the bed and send the energy down to your toes," I said.

"Do you mean touch my toes?"

"No, just think of sending the energy there." She did, and

again they relaxed a little more, but not enough to move with comfort.

I had had an experience of tetany myself, at a time when my body was resisting some kind of excitement. Thinking about what Tracy had told me about her family, I realized that the person she was protecting from her excitement was her mother. "Tracy," I said, "reach out as if you were a small child, and touch your mother's face."

As she did so, feeling herself make contact with her mother's cheeks, the stiffness in her hands dissolved. She did this three or four times, reaching out with both hands. "This is incredible," she said. "It's like something out of a science fiction movie, with aliens who zap people with lightning bolts coming out of their fingers. Each fingertip feels alive, and it's releasing energy."

With her fingers moving again, she told me that she felt drained but ecstatic. "I can't wait for the surgery. We're going to blow everybody's doors off!"

THE LAST SACRIFICE

Tracy was the first patient who told me that her experience with me actually made her look forward to the surgery instead of dreading it, but it was something I would hear many times again. It was, perhaps, the greatest compliment I could possibly receive. It meant that the patients were realizing some previously unacknowledged potential for healing in this brutal and violent experience. It meant that they were focused on transforming the energy of invasion into the energy of creation.

Tracy's surgery was scheduled for three o'clock on the following day, but as is so often the case, there was a long delay, and we didn't get into the operating room until five. Her husband, Robert, seemed withdrawn and frightened.

As Tracy lay on the gurney in the holding area, I held her hand. From time to time tears welled up in her eyes, and I told her that it was all right to be afraid. She admitted that the idea of waking up without her right breast was scaring her. When Dr. Morris came over, Tracy introduced us, telling each how wonderful the other one was. Dr. Morris looked surprised, as if she hadn't known that Tracy had so much faith in her. But because her healing after the lumpectomy, a much more invasive procedure, had gone so much faster than her healing from the original biopsy, Tracy had complete trust in Dr. Morris's skill and care.

I liked Shana Morris even more in person than I had on the phone. She had a warmth and inclusiveness that I had not encountered before in a surgeon. She didn't allow her professional stance to interfere with her natural ebullience and affection for people.

Inside the operating room things went very much as I had described them to Tracy the night before. When Dr. Morris made the initial incision, I sensed in the anesthetized Tracy a terrible sorrow at the prospect of more loss in her life. So I leaned over and told Tracy that giving up her breast was the last sacrifice she would have to make. When I put my hands around the breast specimen before it was sent to be biopsied, it didn't feel energetically like the cancerous tissue I had felt before. Instead of compacted rage, I felt weeping, screaming, and struggling—movement instead of frozen motion. I wondered what this meant. The lymph node specimens were labeled and whisked out of the room to pathology before I had a chance to feel them.

Like Dr. Estabrook, Dr. Morris was extremely careful about preserving all the nerves in the arm from which she took the nodes, pointing them out to me as she did so. I assumed that this was standard practice—until I started working in other cities, where the cavalier attitude about nerve preservation on the part of some of the surgeons I encountered shocked me. In the next sixteen months, with thirty more breast cancer surgeries, I learned that different surgeons doing the same operation are like different musicians playing the same piece. They start and finish in the same place, but that is all.

Tracy did not get back to her room until ten o'clock that night, and although she was longing to go home, Dr. Morris wanted her to stay in the hospital for two more days, until Wednesday. When she and her assistant saw Tracy on Tuesday morning, however, they were both struck by how strong her color was and how good she looked. "My God, you look fantastic," Dr. Morris said, and agreed to take out one of the two drains she had put in to take fluid out of the wounds, and send her home.

That Friday Tracy's friend, Nancy, drove her up to my house for a post-op session. Before we went upstairs to do energy work on the table, Tracy said something harsh and judgmental about herself, and I almost felt her mother standing behind her in the room. I knew that she must have had a great deal of unexpressed anger toward her mother (as did every breast cancer patient I would see), but was not certain what would enable her to release it.

"Tell me more about your relationship with your mother when you were a little girl," I said.

"She was very critical and very controlling," Tracy said, "and I wasn't allowed to play." There was a catch in her throat as she said this. "All the other girls wore pants to school or shorts under their dresses, so they could run around and do handstands and somersaults in the schoolyard and no one would see their underwear. My mother wouldn't let me wear pants or shorts. She thought it wasn't ladylike. And there were two girls at the bus stop who would torture me about it. One would grab my arms, and the other would pull my dress up." Parents so unfeelingly inflict and allow to be inflicted a thousand tiny cruelties on their children—imposing meaningless restraints and rules that do nothing more than assert their authority over an excited and vulnerable little soul. They deny their own pain by passing it along.

"She wouldn't let me go to other kids' houses because she said she 'had to keep an eye on me.' And she wouldn't let me play in our house, or have anyone else over to play, because she said it made too much noise and would disturb my grandparents." Although Tracy said all this in her usual brisk, clipped manner, the feeling in her throat began to throb in her chest. I went over and put my hands on her—one in the center of her chest, just over the thymus gland, and one just opposite, on her back.

"Tracy," I said, "I want you to take a deep breath and, as you exhale, say, 'I want to play.'" She did so in a very small voice, quite unlike her normally assured and assertive tone, and a shudder ran through her body. Hearing this quiet voice, I marveled again at how people to whom anger seems so accessible about a host of things in their everyday lives, have so much trouble attaching anger to the things that have really hurt them.

"Say it again," I told her. She did, in a slightly stronger voice, but tears of helplessness welled up her eyes. "This is not pain," I told her. "This is anger. I want you to stand up, face the wall, visualize your mother on the wall, make fists, and say this as angrily as you can. And take in lots of air. You're going to need it."

"I want to play," she said in a pleading voice.

"Louder," I said. "She can barely hear you. And don't beg."

After a few tries Tracy started to connect with the feeling, and Nancy and I both felt a current of energy moving down her body. "Send the feeling out your eyes," I told her, putting my hands on her pelvis and at the base of her spine, to help draw the energy down. "Now really belt it out," I said, "and send your voice down into the floor, through your genitals, as if you were pushing down and giving birth." She came through with a roar of sound, and suddenly the exercise started to feel very easy.

"I want to *plaaaaaay*!" Tracy screamed. "I want to *plaaaaaaay*!

I want to PLAAAAAAAY!" As with Walter, the energy in the room was completely transformed, and Nancy and I felt a lightness and a tingling in our bodies.

"Look at me, Tracy," I said, and as she turned to do so, a new feeling came up in her. This time it was true pain—the knowledge and valuing of the self—welling up from her chest to her throat to her head. As I moved to hug her, she cried softly and shook, having risked a great deal by defying her mother in this way.

BEING HURT AND KNOWING WHO WE ARE

I realize that my use of the word *pain* in this context requires some explanation, beyond what I said when I first introduced the concept of four basic feelings. When we've been "hurt," either emotionally or physically—when someone violates us, on a physical or emotional level—the normal emotional response is anger. As children, we may have been trained to cry instead of express anger, because crying was more acceptable and may have been modeled for us by our mothers. But the feeling behind the tears is rage. True pain, of the kind Tracy experienced, comes from valuing ourselves, or from feeling valued. We associate it with being hurt because an attack on our vulnerability is what identifies it for us. After Tracy defended herself with her anger, the knowledge of how precious she was came out in the open—the knowledge that what her mother had tried to control and destroy in her, her vulnerable excitement, was actually important and worth defending.

We can also get to a pain feeling by taking in a loving feeling from another person. It's the way we feel when someone else stands up for us or just gives us a hug. It's a feeling of being completely at our own center, at the very core of our being, where loving feeling is received.

Tracy later said of her experience, "It was like opening a trapdoor in my soul. It really worked. And after that, things just kept coming out."

I asked Nancy, who was now beaming a strong loving feeling at Tracy, if she would like to help me do some energy work on her. She agreed, and the three of us went upstairs. When Tracy lay down, I stood at her head and asked Nancy to hold her big toes. Tracy sank into a state of deep relaxation, and I allowed energy to flow through my hands into her head, her throat, her chest, and especially the site of the surgery. Nancy, to her surprise, also went into a light trance; she told us at the end of the session that images of Tracy as a child came to her. Very powerful waves of energy had flowed from Tracy's body into her hands. Tracy had felt both energized and relaxed.

The place where the drainage tube emerged from Tracy's body had been numb since the surgery, but when she got home that afternoon and was walking the dog, sensation in the area "switched itself on," as she called me very excitedly that evening to tell me. She saw Dr. Morris the following Tuesday, eight days after the surgery. Her healing had proceeded so rapidly that Dr. Morris had to dig into her flesh to get out the stitches, because she had healed right over them.

Standing Up to the System

The pathology report revealed that no cancer had existed in the breast—that, in essence, a perfectly healthy breast had been removed from Tracy's body. This explained to me why I'd felt no compacted rage in the tissue sample. Tracy had expected Dr. Morris to be excited about this news, but again she was disappointed. Since four of the thirteen lymph nodes removed from her arm were positive, Dr. Morris wanted her to have chemotherapy and radiation. Tracy refused, but she agreed, at Dr. Morris's urging, to talk to an oncologist.

Tracy liked Anne Silver, the oncologist, a great deal, although she was not pleased with Dr. Silver's answers to her questions. "If I do all this," Tracy asked, "if I do the chemo, which you admit is poison, eight treatments, one every three weeks, with nausea, weakness, and my hair falling out, followed by radiation, or tamoxifen, which will increase my chances of getting uterine cancer and which I have to take for the rest of my life—if I do all this and ask you at the end of it, 'Am I going to be okay?' would you tell me, 'We don't know'?"

"Yes, I would," said Dr. Silver.

"And if I ask you if the cancer has spread, and where it has spread to, would you say, 'I don't know'?"

"Yes," said Dr. Silver.

"And I would have to wait ten or fifteen years to know if I'm going to be okay?"

"That's also true."

"So bottom line, what's the benefit?" Tracy asked.

"Statistics show that it reduces the risk of recurrence thirty percent," Dr. Silver said. Tracy would later find this figure refuted in a book written by another physician on adjunctive cancer therapies, which cited statistics showing that for stage two breast cancer, chemo and radiation increase the chances for survival by only 7 percent.

"What about your patients who have decided not to do chemo or radiation?" Tracy asked. "What do you know about their survival rates?" Dr. Silver admitted that she never hears from them and so doesn't know what has happened to them. Tracy was appalled that she was recommending a treatment so drastic in its side effects, without any firsthand knowledge of what happens to people who decide to forgo it.

Many months later I found myself visiting a surgeon who was very upset about a patient who was unwilling to follow her mastectomy with chemo and radiation. "Why are you so upset?" I asked.

"Because she's going to die," the surgeon replied.

"Suppose she does the chemo and radiation, and then she dies? Would you still be upset?"

"No," she responded, an answer that sent me reeling, "because we all know that cancer is a fatal disease."

I spent a lot of time thinking about this conversation and about why these two very dangerous and virulent treatments were the best the medical establishment had been able to come up with in the "war on cancer." Why the enchantment with poisoning and burning? Particularly in so many cases where no clear data demonstrate that these treatments extend life? I also wondered about the disease itself. The only cells that grow as fast as cancer cells are fetal cells. Why, I wondered, would a part of the body want to go back to that very early moment in its development? What was it trying to learn about, to get right this time, to tell us, or to express?

Tracy continued to resist pressure from both her family and her physicians, one of whom called her "crazy" and another "in denial," and to work on herself with jin shin jitsu. I was so impressed with both her courage and her devotion to the treatment that I regularly suggested to other breast cancer patients that they talk to her and go for treatments with her when possible. A couple of them ended up taking the training.

Although the surgeries performed to treat breast cancer are much less challenging than cardiac surgeries and are less interesting in terms of both anatomy and physiology, I found a great deal of relief at being able to move out of the world of cardiac surgery. For one thing, it bothered me that their heavy research and surgery loads left the cardiac surgeons at Columbia so little time to spend with each patient. After surgery, the patients were turned over to the cardiologists, while the surgeons moved on to their next heroic encounter with life and death. In addition, there was at times a certain gender amnesia in cardiac surgery. Once I heard a resident talk about reperfusing (putting blood back into) "his heart," but it was a woman on the table.

"Uh, 'her' heart," I said.

"Oh yes, yes, of course."

A week later a similar incident happened, this time with an attending surgeon, and I didn't bother to correct him.

By now I was convinced that repeated emotional distress and abuse, starting very early on in life and usually ignored or denied by the patient, are a key factor in weakening the body and making it vulnerable to chronic disease. I looked around at all the paraphernalia that made possible this so-called medical miracle of patching and replacing hearts, and I thought of the hundreds of thousands of dollars it represented, multiplied by thousands of operating rooms all around the country. How miraculous, indeed, that we could create so much technology and spend so much money in order not to get to a feeling. And how few and bold are patients like Tracy, who are willing to back off from the technology and explore the feeling wisdom of their bodies.

Chapter Nine

REBUILDING THE BODY, RECONSTRUCTING THE PAST

I once saw a photograph on a magazine cover of a woman with a flat chest and a mastectomy scar and thought she looked quite beautiful. In spite of what some would consider her disfigurement, she was giving off a completely intact sexual feeling, and it was compellingly attractive. My feelings to the contrary, however, most women under fifty do decide to have their absent breasts "reconstructed." I have heard plastic surgeons claim—perhaps a little defensively—that this procedure "completes" a woman's healing from her disease.

Despite the physical discomfort that attends all of the various surgeries used to recreate breasts on female bodies, Americans generally seem to believe that looking good is more important than feeling good. This is not to say that I disapprove of plastic surgery of any kind, any more than I disapprove of expensive clothes, tattooing, makeup, or body building. But like everything else we do to alter our appearance, breast reconstruction has many layers of meaning, and profound healing can occur when all of these are explored.

The first reconstructive surgery I worked on was another case of Shana Morris's. Andrea was a slender, stylish woman in her early forties who lived in a high-ceilinged loft in the wholesale flower district of Manhattan.

She was a freelance writer and once had been married to a very successful but alcoholic musician. She thought that there might be some correlation between the onset of her breast cancer and the disintegration of her marriage. Her father, she told me, was also an alcoholic. So many of the breast cancer patients I saw had had at least one alcoholic parent that I was surprised that no one had collected statistics or studied a possible correlation. Andrea had a nine-year-old daughter whom she adored, and she worried intensely about the effect the disease was having on her. She was concerned that Georgina would have to take care of her instead of the other way around, and she feared both the strain it would put on her and the resentment it might create in her daughter.

Andrea clearly needed nurturing desperately. I tried to assure her that allowing her daughter to care for her would be a gift to the girl. "Didn't you have a desire to protect and take care of your mother?" I asked. She sighed. "And didn't you want, more than anything else, for her to take in and acknowledge your love and your caring?" I felt pain welling up in her and saw tears coming into her eyes.

More than anything else, breast cancer appears to me to be about this tortured relationship between mother and daughter. The women I have worked with seem nurturing themselves, but time after time a sense of their mothers' bitter feeling about the pregnancy, the state of the marriage at the time of conception, or the responsibility of having to care for a child when they felt so uncared for themselves came through. When I mentioned this to a woman who worked at SHARE, a breast cancer support organization, she told me that the saddest thing was that the patients sometimes expected that the onset of the disease would somehow change this situation—that their mothers would suddenly fly to their sides, full of tenderness, understanding, and caring. In some cases it did happen, but the disappointment when it didn't was devastating. It was perhaps even more upsetting when the mother did arrive and succeeded once more in putting herself at the center of concern, instead of her daughter.

Somehow this bitterness about nurturing is transferred to the daughter, who carries it inside her own breast. Just how this psychological transition weakens tissue or turns on those genes that make possible cancerous growth, was not clear to me. I just knew that stories of maternal abuse, neglect, narcissism, and resentment were just too common for their relationship to this disease to be ignored.

FEELINGS AND DNA

Perhaps breast cancer is the effect of the withheld rage that these women are feeling. Since anger has the same energetic quality as acceleration, or gravity, it has the power to distort space and bend electromagnetic waves, as Einstein described in his theory of relativity. Therefore anger held in the cells could affect the electromagnetic bonds in DNA chains. Reba Goodman, at Columbia, has demonstrated in her laboratory (much to the discomfort of the power companies) that the electrochemical bonds in DNA molecules are so delicate that very low-level electromagnetic frequencies can alter that molecular structure. So, I posited, what was damaging the DNA and triggering the cancerous growth could either be the energy of the anger, or the energy of the fear constraining the anger, which is itself an electromagnetic force.

Julie
Motz

168

But why would such energy alter the DNA in this very particular way, turning ordinary cells into undifferentiated, fast-growing ones like those of a human embryo? Since the earliest nurturing is the nurturing of the conceptus inside the womb, did the impotent rage go back to that period? Could the problem be, not that normal breast tissue was being converted, but that one or two cells from that period had never developed into mature breast tissue and were now suddenly triggered into rampant growth?

Andrea, a lean, very health-conscious woman with a chest almost as flat as a dancer's, had elected to have tram-flap reconstruction done immediately following her mastectomy. This meant that when the general surgeon finished removing Andrea's breast, a plastic surgeon would take over in the OR and rebuild the breast from tissue from Andrea's lower abdomen. An incision would be made below the navel and above the pubic bone, and a wedge of flesh, with one of the two ricutus muscles that support the stomach area still attached, would be tunneled up under the skin of the abdomen and the chest and pushed out through the hole of the mastectomy incision to form a breast. Later, some skin at the center would be puckered up to form a nipple, and the appropriate colors tattooed on. Although this procedure would deprive the abdomen of half of its normal support, it was necessary to leave the ricutus muscle attached in order to provide the blood supply for the transposed lower abdominal tissue.

For women who are overweight, the operation has the double advantage of giving them a new breast and removing an unsightly bulge, but this was not the case with Andrea, so her choice surprised me. I did not ask her why she had elected to have this particular surgery, which would leave her stomach area with only half its normal support. A highly intelligent and well-informed woman, I assumed she knew what the downside was. I had no desire to challenge her or to add to her discomfort or insecurity about what she was about to undergo. Perhaps the trauma of the divorce had left her feeling that going out into the world one-breasted would just be unacceptable.

I did some energy work at her head and feet to relax her, then took her through the surgery step by step. We parted with a warm hug and met again a few days later at the hospital.

As is routine with most surgeries, the anesthesiologist met Andrea in the holding area outside the operating room to ask her a series of questions, including what medications she was allergic to, if there was any bridge work in her mouth that had to be removed, and if she had had any previous surgery. "I had an abortion," she said, apparently without feeling—except that I could sense a pain ripping through her uterus. I knew from our previous session that she had also had a miscarriage, and I was surprised that she hadn't mentioned the abortion to me as well. Perhaps she had decided, as so many women do, to treat it as nothing important in her life.

In the operating room I felt a great deal of panic in her as the breathing tube was pushed down her immobilized throat. I saw her as a small child in a hospital bed and remembered a story she told about being left alone in the hospital after a pediatric tonsillectomy. As the surgeon worked to remove Andrea's breast, I felt a great deal of anguish in it about her daughter. I told her that Georgina completely experienced all her love, and the anguish eased. I felt sorrow and weeping in the excised breast tissue when I put my hands around the specimen, and rage in the lymph nodes.

A fourth-year medical student had "scrubbed in" (washed her hands up to the elbows in sterilizing soap and put on sterile gloves and a sterile gown) and was assisting Dr. Morris for part of the surgery. Close to the end of the mastectomy, an intern, also scrubbed, came into the operating room and suggested to the medical student that she go have lunch. The student clearly was upset at being "bumped" in this manner, but the hierarchy was clear, and she had no choice.

As the plastic surgeon began to work, I observed that the incision he made in Andrea's lower abdomen was directly over her uterus and her ovaries. Fear and pain swept through her body, and I felt her experiencing memories of both the abortion and the miscarriage, along with all her mother's conflicted feelings about having children. I told her to give that feeling back to her mother, that she did not have to carry it in her body any longer. I also told her that it was time to release the spirits of those two lost children and let them leave her energy field with complete love and with the knowledge that they would incarnate in another place and at another time that would be right for them. I also told her that if she had kept those children, she would have had no room in her life for Georgina, whom she loved so much.

The plastic surgeon commented on how very small her breasts were—so small, in fact, that it was hard to shape a small enough section from her abdomen to get the right size. I understood now, however, why Andrea had elected this procedure: she needed to reactivate all the feelings held in her reproductive organs and find some way at least to experience if not to release them. It occurred to me for the first time that perhaps people come into surgery for just this reason: that the reactivation of old trauma is not just an unfortunate side effect but a straining of the body to heal on every level. So perhaps my presence in the operating room was part of some inevitable evolution in humanity's continuing struggle to come to terms with its pain. Perhaps the forces that had conspired to put me here, in the presence of the ultimate vulnerability and the ultimate transgression, had little to do with my own curiosity and ambition. Sooner or later someone was destined to hear the soul's cry from the body: "Here I am, showing you my deepest wounds. Watch, feel, and listen—and heal me by telling me what you witness, and by holding it out to me with love." It just happened to be me.

By now the medical student was back, scrubbed in again but simply observing at the side of the table. Andrea was withdrawing, and the surgeon seemed to be working at a slower pace—in fact, we were about half an hour behind schedule. I got an image of a child crawling around on the floor, feeling bereft, being ignored by some male figure who was supposed to be taking care of her. My eyes were drawn to the medical student: hidden rage at being stuck in this impotent position was oozing out from her, affecting everyone in the room. Although there was nothing I could comfortably say, I felt that I had to protect Andrea by getting the student out of the room. I focused my attention on the student and silently sent the message "I despise you for what you're doing, and I want you out of the operating room." About a minute later, to my surprise and relief, she announced that she had to go, ripped off her gloves and gown, and left.

A few days later I saw Andrea in the hospital for a post-op session. As was always the case with these surgeries, she had a great deal of tightness in the front of her body, and she couldn't completely straighten up because of the reversed muscle. She told me, however, that everyone had remarked on how good she looked and how much energy she had. I told her what I had experienced during the surgery, leaving out the part about the medical student. Nor did I share with her my conviction that she had elected this surgery in order to activate certain memories and feelings. But she received the information I gave her about those feelings and memories with great interest, and she seemed to be on a path of healing and transformation. I finished my session with her by placing a hand over each of her breasts—old and new—and suggesting to the new one that it learn, vibrationally, from the other, how to be a breast. As I did this, I felt a settling down in Andrea's chest.

This was the first time I had worked with a plastic surgeon, and it made me think about the whole process of reshaping and reconstructing the body to fit our image of how we're supposed to look. Was it really all about releasing feelings held in the flesh? Bonnie Cohen had said that a baby first finds its mother's breast by bobbing after it with its nose; were all those "nose jobs," so popular as sixteenth-birthday presents when I was growing up, really about trying to reconfigure that very early connection? Did they imagine that with a different nose their mother would accept groping for their love more easily?

The Roots of Disease

A few months later I gave a talk at the annual conference of the International Society for the Study of Subtle Energy and Energy Medicine in Boulder. This had always been a favorite conference of mine, both because of the simple clean energy that Boulder, nestled against the Rockies, exudes, and because of the bright, earnest, like-minded people who gather here for the three-day event. My talk was about my work in surgery, and a number of people came up to me afterward with questions and comments.

Hanging back a little from the others was a tall, lean, square-jawed woman who finally approached me rather shyly after the others had left. As she talked to me, she was wringing her hands, which struck me as childlike, as if she were comforting herself with the contact. She told me that she was a physician from the Midwest and that she was about to have plastic surgery on her face. She was going to have the skin around her face tightened. It looked perfectly normal to me, and my look of surprise must have been evident, because she hastened to explain that her husband had left her the year before and that she had lost a lot of weight as a result.

She then volunteered that her brother had offered to come and take her home from the hospital. Instinctively, I put my left hand out and held it just over her right jaw. I felt a sharp, shooting pain. "What happened to your face?" I asked.

"My brother broke my jaw when I was four," she told me.

"Well, all the feelings you have about it are still in there, and

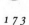

I guarantee that they will come up when you go in for the surgery. I really suggest that you try to get to them before that."

"I've forgiven my brother, of course," she said.

"Yes, but your face hasn't. And now you can't get angry at him because he's the one who's going to be taking care of you." She stared at me, blankly at first—and then I felt it sink into her. "Whatever your husband did to you, I suspect, mirrored something that some man in your family did much earlier. You don't have to confront your brother about it, because it isn't about your relationship with him anymore. But I think you need to go into the feeling in your jaw and let some of that rage out before the surgery."

She called me six weeks later to tell me that her recovery from the surgery had been remarkably swift, astonishing her surgeon and delighting her friends. She was using herbs and energy work to help speed the process. I didn't ask her about her anger toward her brother, but she told me that she had been talking to her face, and I sensed a calmness in her that had not been there before.

Some time after this I talked to Loren Eskenazi, a very talented plastic surgeon from San Francisco with a long-standing interest in alternative medicine. She told me that it very often takes people a number of weeks before they can actually "own" the changes she creates for them. With a healer in the OR consciously processing whatever feelings were in the tissue, we speculated, this might happen much faster. Dr. Eskenazi also bemoaned the fact that psychological dissatisfactions often remain even after the physical flaws have been removed. I told her about my vision of surgery in which both levels of healing are accomplished, and she was the first surgeon with whom I spoke who openly embraced this idea.

The more deeply I got into surgery, the more strongly this idea of total healing absorbed me. I had a growing sense that little in my own life was accidental—that I was bringing things across my path in an effort to learn things about myself that I couldn't learn in any other way, and that every cell in my body was a full participant in this learning process. The same, I believe, is true for everyone. Then what is each patient, each surgeon, each anesthesiologist, and each OR nurse and technician trying to learn when they come together? And what are we, as a culture, trying to dramatize for ourselves in these situations?

It became more and more apparent to me that we have violent medicine because we have a violent society, and that the root of this violence is the cruelty and humiliation inflicted upon children by their parents. Disease is facilitated by the violence of childhood, and we can think of healing only in terms of matching this violence. That is why we have a "war" on cancer, and why surgeons see themselves as heroes on a bloody battlefield, dashing in to save lives. It is probably why we do not practice a great deal more preventive medicine.

Gradually, I came to see all disease as an attempt by the body to call us back to earlier wounds and to jolt us into dealing with them. I also saw the cures we have created as a critical part of reenacting these early dramas.

DENIAL

I did ten breast cancer surgeries in the metropolitan New York area, at five different hospitals. In each case the woman had had both recent turmoil and ancient tragedy in her life. In each case she had a sense of urgency about changing her life, confusion about how to do this, and often anger at outside forces that seemed to be preventing the change. At times, too, they were in profound denial.

Grace was an attractive Afro-American woman in her late thirties with a rambunctious preteen daughter and no husband around to share the responsibility. A paralegal at a large law firm, she was very concerned that if her employers found out about her breast cancer, it would somehow affect her position there. A

Hands
of
Life

175

vegetarian and a meditator who had spent time in a yoga ashram, she was shocked and disappointed when a troubling mammogram, followed by a biopsy, pointed to the need for surgery. "I've done everything right!" she wailed when she came to see me. "I don't understand how this could be happening to me."

As she told me about her life, anger at her mother, who was both controlling and neglectful, came up. Still, she insisted that there had been nothing really abusive about her childhood. Nonetheless, when I suggested she do an anger exercise toward her mother (visualizing her image on the wall and shouting "liar" at her), she agreed and succeeded in letting go with a few terrific angry blasts that brought tears of relief and self-acknowledgment to her eyes.

A few days later, just before the surgery, she called me. "I have to tell you something," she said. "When you suggested that I might have had an abusive childhood and that some feelings about that could be weakening my body, I thought you were crazy. And then lying in bed that night I remembered that my father used to sit at the dinner table every night drinking—getting drunker and drunker as the meal went on—with a gun in his hand. He would threaten to shoot my mother if she didn't shut up and stop her nagging. I sat there silently begging her to just shut up so he wouldn't kill her. As soon as dinner was over, I would run upstairs to my room and lie on the bed, planning how I would escape from the house through my window if he shot her and came after me. I lived in terror. But isn't it funny, my first response when you asked the question was 'No, no, there wasn't any abuse in my family.'"

Actually, I told her, this kind of self-deception is quite common, and it was the reason her body was holding the terror for her.

Her quick recovery from the surgery pleased her, but she locked horns with her surgeon some months later, when she was still refusing to do the chemotherapy that had been recommended. Eventually the surgeon, who had at first told her she would support her in whatever choice she made about follow-up treatment, told her that she couldn't live with her decision to forgo the chemo and told her to find another surgeon.

Partly because of her commitment to self-healing and partly because she was afraid to take too much time off from work, Grace continued with her own regimen of herbs, diet, prayer, meditation, and therapy. When I spoke to her almost two years later, she told me that she was feeling terrific, although she would always live in the shadow of knowing that the disease could return.

THE WEAPONS OF THE WEAK

Wendy, who came to me after her surgery, told me that she knew exactly when the cancer had first started attacking her body. "It was six years ago, when my husband had his first and only affair in the history of our marriage. We both realized that it was all about an identity crisis he was having around his work. I was hurt at first, but he was extremely sorry about it, and I forgave him completely." She said she had also forgiven her mother, who had never wanted her and had left her, as a small child, alone by an open fire with no grate on it. She had fallen into the fire and been taken to the hospital with terrible disfiguring third-degree burns all over her body and her face, which multiple plastic surgeries had not completely restored. Her mother had also forced this extremely bright and intellectually astute girl to leave school to go to work, at a time when teachers were urging her to try for a scholarship to a university.

Wendy told me very emphatically that she did not want to be angry at anyone—but she was very angry at the disease, which had spread from her breast to her lung and was attacking her at a time when she and her husband, now retired, had planned to do nothing but enjoy themselves. She made a modest stab at modifying her diet, took all kinds of supplements, herbs, and teas, and put herself through every course of chemotherapy her doctors suggested, but she got weaker each time. The radiation they gave her resulted in terrible, painful burns, convincing me that she was determined to relive all the abuse and neglect of her childhood rather than become angry about it. I was again struck by the idea that not only can the symptoms of disease recapitulate old trauma, but that the very cures people select, both individually and collectively, as a culture, can do the same thing.

Wendy's husband, Harold, who truly adored her, suffered terribly during the whole process. I finally decided that as much as she loved him, she had not been able to truly forgive him for his betrayal, because he was the one and only person in her life she had trusted. Nor could she get angry at him and admit how deeply she felt the pain he had caused her. All she could do was fight with what T. S. Eliot called "the weapons of the weak / which [are] too violent"—the weapons of self-destruction. By hurting herself, she would hurt him—and thereby make him pay for his infidelity.

Several months later I learned that Wendy had died, and a terrible sense of failure came over me. What would have happened, I wondered, if I had just said, "Look, this is all happening because you're determined to make Harold pay for the affair by suffering through your sickness and your death? He's trapped, not being able to get angry at you for leaving him, just as you felt both abandoned and impotent when he had the affair." My judgment call at the time was that she wouldn't have been open to the information—but suppose I was wrong? Or even if I was right, couldn't I have found some way to lead her to the insight? After all, isn't that what a healer's job is all about—making the patient feel safe enough to take in love and information?

I tried to tell myself that if someone wants to take revenge on a mate by dying instead of getting angry, that's fine. But in my heart I didn't believe it. I had worshipped too long at the altar of the emotions to abandon my creed. My underlying, secret goal remained to make the world safe for feelings. I had become a healer because physical distress often forces upon people the recognition of the need for change on a feeling level. Emotional change, even for relatively healthy people, often requires a physical approach. But unless the emotional change occurred as well, the work of physical healing, just making people feel better, was empty and unsatisfying for me.

SYMPTOMS AND MEMORY

The idea that all disease represents some kind of regression came to me first not through surgery but from my fascination with neurological disorders. A man in one of Bonnie Cohen's workshops had told us he had tried out her technique of moving from different tissues and fluids with his mother, who had Parkinson's disease. When he suggested that she try to move from her synovial fluid (the fluid that lubricates the joints), he said that her otherwise jerky movements had become perfectly smooth and continuous.

The idea fascinated me that even in a diseased state the body holds a memory of health in certain cells and can summon it up to override the disease. I had a chance to try this out for myself when a cardiac patient I was preparing for her surgery told me that she had a tremor in her legs from Parkinson's. I asked her to try to move one of her legs from each of the four basic tissues (nerves, muscles, bones, and marrow), and then from the fluids (cerebrospinal, blood, lymph, and synovial). Sure enough, when she got to synovial fluid, the movement became easy and smooth. It was also smooth moving from bone marrow.

The jerkiness of her disease, I realized, came from some problem in nerve transmission—in emotional terms, some distortion of her fear feeling. When she moved from bone marrow or synovial fluid, she was moving from her loving feeling instead.

A couple of months later, I had another opportunity to work with a Parkinson's patient, although things went in a direction I had not anticipated. A cardiac patient told me that his wife, Jane, who was a nurse, had Parkinson's. I offered to do an energy session with her in return for just finding out more about the disease. When I got to their home in suburban Connecticut, she was waiting for me, along with a friend who shared some of her deeply held religious convictions and was involved in a Bible study course with her. They were both very gentle and pleasant-looking women in their late fifties. Jane was quite slender and a little stooped, while Mary was tall and plump.

Jane explained to me that Mary was very interested in healing and had asked if she could be present at the session. "Fine," I said. "In fact, if she likes, she can help." Mary laughed shyly and demurred.

"I really don't know very much about this disease," I told Jane. "I don't even know what all its symptoms are. So why don't you start by telling me what about it troubles you the most?"

"Well," she said with a sad, apologetic smile, "it's the way I walk."

"Could you show me?" I asked. She got up off the couch and shuffled across the living room, taking small, very hesitant steps. "You look like a toddler," I said spontaneously. She turned her head and smiled at me, a big, wide, almost conspiratorial grin, and I felt a wave of energy running down her spine.

Mary had a surprised expression on her face and leaned back, as if something had caught her off balance. "Did you feel that release of energy down her back?" I asked. She nodded.

I got up, and started to do the shuffling walk myself, just to get the feel of it. "Okay," I said, "I'd like you to do the walk again, Jane, but there's one thing I'd like you to add. I want you to look up as you do it, as if you were really one and a half or two and everybody around you were taller than you are." I demonstrated this for a few steps and could feel in my own body a kind of sweet, delicious energy, as well as a sadness.

Obediently, Jane did the walk with her head tilted up. Another flood of energy came down her spine, and a lightness seemed to take over her whole being.

When she sat down I told her, "Look, I don't know much about this disease, but symptomatically it seems to be taking you back to a time when you were very young and walked in just this way. You also seemed to be very happy then. So what I want to know is, what happened at just that time to interrupt this feeling?"

"When I was one and a half, my mother had another baby," Jane said without missing a beat, as if she had been waiting for someone to ask. "My little brother was born, and after that she ignored me."

"Okay," I said, "I want you to get up again and do the walk again, holding your head tilted up. But this time I want you to say 'I want to be the baby!' over and over again."

Jane got up and started to do her shuffle, head tilted up as if looking at her mother. "I want to be the baby," she said. "I want to be the baby! I want to be the baaaaby!" Her spine became very straight, her walk much faster and more aggressive, and her voice reached a decibel level I would hardly have thought possible a few moments before. It was clear to me that this forbidden rage was somehow at the core of her disease—a rage that her family upbringing and religious conviction did not give her permission to express.

Later, when I was doing some research about cocaine addiction and trying to understand the correlations between the drug's effect on neurotransmitters and the emotions it blocked, I went into my body to feel the energy of each of the four major ones: norepinephrine, dopamine, acetylcholine, and serotonin. I realized that they correspond, in turn, to fear, anger, pain, and love. Of the four basic neurotransmitters, dopamine is the one that carries anger. Parkinson's patients suffer from a dopamine deficiency in the brain.

Neurotransmitter	Feeling
Norepinephrine	Fear
Dopamine	Anger
Acetylcholine	Pain
Serotonin	Love

Clearly, the symptom of Parkinson's carries the meaning of the disease. It had taken Jane back to a time when her happiness was first ruptured. I believed it would keep her there, unless she became comfortable in expressing her anger at that rupture. I explained this to her and asked her if she would like to do an exercise to focus that anger. She declined but thanked me for the work we'd done. Her refusal did not surprise me. Every social norm we have supports the suppression of anger, except in war and in sports—activities only recently open to women.

Chapter Ten

MUSCLES AND NERVES

Waiting to meet with Bennett Stein, Columbia's chief of neurosurgery, I had come across a newsletter for patients with ALS
(amyotrophic lateral sclerosis), a disease in which nerves and
muscles degenerate, finally to the point where the diaphragm
and the digestive tract no longer work and the patient dies. To
date, there is no known cure for "Lou Gehrig's disease," as it is
also called, and the diagnosis is often regarded as a death sentence, albeit a sometimes slow-approaching one. What caught
my attention in the newsletter was the announcement that the
next ALS patients' monthly meeting would feature a presenta-
tion about music therapy.

To see anything alternative being presented to any group of
patients at Columbia was so exciting and so startling that I got
in touch with the people running this group. A short game of
telephone tag eventually brought me to the small paper-flooded
office of Peregrine Murphy and Maura Del Bene, a social
worker and a nurse (respectively) who ran the program and pro-

duced the newsletter. I was immediately struck by their un-abashed warmth for their patients. I told them quite frankly that I'd never worked with an ALS patient but had a hunch that I might be able to help and would like to try.

I left them some material about my work in surgery, and about a month later I got a call from a woman who introduced herself as "Mr. King's secretary." She told me that her boss had been given my name by Maura Del Bene and would like to set up an appointment.

The man whose driver delivered him to my door a few days later was a delightful set of contradictions. With a recently con-firmed diagnosis of ALS, Maurice King had plunged into a number of alternative treatments, including acupuncture, vita-mins and supplements, and massage, and he had also gotten himself included in a clinical trial of a neurotrophic (nerve growth) factor drug. Yet he had no thought of giving up either cigarettes or bourbon and was most concerned about what the disease would do to his golf score. He was already having some trouble walking, with a marked weakness and a "drop foot" (in-ability to flex the ankle) in one leg.

The retired owner of a very successful manufacturing firm, with a quick wit and a sense of self-deprecating irony, Maurice did not seem to feel any resentment about what was happening to him. In fact, he remarked that he was a lot more cheerful about it than his doctors. In my session with him I did a stan-dard energy chelation, with a focus on his head and his left leg, the one that had started to fail him and that felt much less en-ergized than his right. He felt calm, relaxed, and buoyant after the treatment, but walking was only slightly easier. He asked me, with that complete trust that always surprises me in patients, if I thought he should see me again, and how often.

"Why don't you go home and see how you feel, then call me if you want to come back again? I have no idea right now if this is helping, but perhaps your body will tell you. And I'd like to read any literature you have on that neurotrophic factor they're giving you in the trial." A couple of days later a packet of material arrived, and I started to read and to make calls, first to the people running the trial in Florida and then to the manufacturers of the medication.

The popular wisdom about ALS is that it is a nerve disease. Nerves that innervate muscle, for some reason that no one can determine, start to die. Then the muscles atrophy. Some instinct, however, told me that this was not the correct order of things—that it is in the muscles where the disease begins. When I read King's literature, a bell went off in my head. The neurotrophic factor they were using in the trial was initially expressed in the muscle and then transmitted to the nerve. So, following this model, it would be the muscle that failed to stimulate the nerve, then the nerve would die and then the muscle would atrophy.

CELLULAR COMMUNICATION

I called Bonnie Cohen to discuss this idea with her. She had never worked with an ALS patient, but she asked me to send her the literature on the drug. Although she was very busy teaching and her work with private patients was largely restricted to infants and children, she agreed that if Maurice would make the trip up to Amherst, Massachusetts, where she lived, she would see him.

Maurice came for another session a couple of weeks later, and I convinced him to go see Bonnie with me and with my friend Michelle, who wanted to observe. A couple weeks later we met Maurice and his driver in the parking lot of a shopping mall to make the trip. Both men graciously accommodated our presence in the car by not smoking. Michelle sat in front with the driver, while I was in back, next to Maurice. Ever the pragmatist, I decided that we could make use of some of the driving time by doing healing work. Consequently I asked Maurice to stretch his left leg out through the space between the front seats so Michelle could reach it. I leaned across his body and put my hand on his liver, hoping to get to some clues about his hidden anger.

I got an image of a tall, gawky adolescent, and the number fourteen came into my mind, as if someone had just whispered it inside my brain. "What happened when you were fourteen?" I asked Maurice.

"My parents made me switch schools and skip a grade," he said. "I would have been varsity basketball if I'd stayed where I was. But at the new school I didn't make the team." There was just a hint of sadness in his voice and a tightening in his chest as he said this. I moved my hands so that one was in the middle of his chest and the other in the middle of his back.

"Somehow your leg, the very one that seems to be failing you, is remembering this," I said. *And how many other sorrows?* I wondered. Maurice had told me that his mother was a terrific sportswoman but didn't have a lot of time for him. I wondered how she felt about the pregnancy. I was also struck by the fact that this information had not come out when I was working on Maurice before, and I gave credit to Michelle's presence and the loving feeling she was putting out for creating the safety that had allowed Maurice's body to speak to me in this way.

If Maurice had shown any interest in giving up cigarettes, I might have raised that issue through the heaviness in his lungs that I felt between my hands, but I thought it would be counterproductive at that point.

Bonnie Cohen lives in an unpretentious house on the outskirts of Amherst. She asked Maurice to lie down on the floor, and then she put a hand on each leg, just above the ankle. "I'm trying to feel down to the level where the energy is the same on both sides," she explained. Then she took a deep breath. "The problem is in the repair cells in the muscles. We have to go to a level below that, where there's the same healthy flow in the left leg as in the right." She invited Michelle and me to put our hands on Maurice and go to that place in his muscle tissue with her. We did so, seated on either side of him with our hands on his legs. I could feel my hands sinking in (while they were actually resting quite lightly on his left leg), until they seemed to reach a place where there was a very strong energy flow, connecting me to both Bonnie and Michelle. We stayed this way for about fifteen minutes, allowing Maurice's body to also focus its attention at the level of these cells.

"What's been happening," Bonnie told him, "is that the nervous system has been taking an unhealthy pattern in the muscle, copying it, and carrying it to other muscles. We want the nervous system to start copying and spreading a healthy pattern instead. I can't tell you why the muscle went into this pattern in the first place. For that, you'll have to go back into your own history."

She then asked Maurice to sit up and put a ridged rubber ball, about four inches in diameter, under his left foot. She asked him to roll his foot—the one with the ankle he couldn't flex— over the ball, moving it away from him, then pulling it back toward him. He did this with some difficulty. Then Bonnie took his foot in her hand and flexed the ankle, moving the toes up toward the shin very slowly. "I'm showing you how to move your foot just from the muscle," she said, "not from the nerve. Can you feel the difference?" Maurice was uncertain at first. "Now I'll show you movement from the nerve," she said, moving it more quickly and lightly this time.

Bonnie does this by going to the tissue in her own body she wants the movement to come from, then communicating that movement vibrationally to the body of the person she is touching. As she worked with Maurice, trying to get him to distinguish between movement through the nerves—where the nerves were instructing the muscles to move—and movement that originated in the muscle itself, I speculated about how such movement might be possible.

"Because voluntary muscles can twitch without an instruction from the brain to 'move,' we know that they are capable of moving independently of their nerves," Bonnie said. "This is the mind of the body at work." This idea correlated completely with my own observation that consciousness exists in every cell. But the mechanism by which we access and contact this consciousness still intrigued me. Did a chemical message come from the brain through the bloodstream and into the cells, bypassing the nervous system? But the action appeared to be too quick for that—virtually simultaneous with the intention. Was there, instead, a vibrational message that originated in the energy field and communicated directly to the cells? If so, how did this communication take place?

One possible explanation was given to me a year later by Bruce Lipton, a renegade molecular biologist who had left Stanford for a tiny converted garage with a spectacular view south of San Francisco, to write about his ideas and teach the biological basis of energy healing to chiropractic students.

Bruce was one of the first people to introduce the idea that the "brain" and, indeed, the whole "nervous system" of a cell lie in the cell membrane, not in its nucleus. If you remove the nucleus, he observed, the cell can survive. But if you destroy the membrane, it dies. Moreover, it is the proteins on the membrane surface that determine what information as well as what nourishment passes into the cell.

These proteins communicate to transport proteins within the cell by shape-shifting, which occurs as the result of changes in polarization at the ends of the proteins' molecular chain. The changes in polarization (from a positive to a negative electrical charge, or vice versa), Bruce pointed out, could occur through a chemical interaction or from low-level electromagnetic waves, of the kind a strong emotion, a powerful thought, or energy flowing from a healer's hands might produce.

The other possibility is that thought itself is actually a de Broglie wave and interacts directly with matter, altering its vibration.

Bonnie did succeed in getting Maurice to feel the difference between the two kinds of movements. With her hands on his foot and his ankle, he flexed the foot himself—something he hadn't been able to do for six months. She suggested that he practice rolling the ball under his foot, moving from the muscle itself, in the hope that the nerves would pick up this pattern of health and begin to convey it to the rest of the leg.

Bonnie has had extraordinary success working with neurologically damaged children, especially infants whom no one else is willing or able to help. With these children she repatterns the nervous system and the brain through movement—having them learn through the muscles, much as she was doing with Maurice. How strenuously Maurice would pursue this approach, however, was uncertain. He got up and walked around Bonnie's studio, delighted with the way his ankle now seemed to work and the new strength in his leg.

On the way home we decided to stop at a toy store and buy some of the balls, which Michelle and I were also eager to practice with. The next time I had a session with Maurice, he told me that he had sold his apartment in New York and that he and his wife were moving to southern California. He had had trouble, on his own, doing the work with the ball and feeling the difference that Bonnie had shown him. The "drop foot" had come back, and he was feeling somewhat discouraged. Sensing a tiny chink in his armor of cheerfulness, I asked him if he felt angry about what was happening to him. "Yes," he said, "especially when I think about my golf!"

"That's a start," I said. I had him stand up and do the anger exercise that I had taken Walter through—facing the wall, making fists, and saying with as much feeling as possible, "I'm angry." In spite of feeling foolish initially, he did manage to connect to his anger a couple of times and then, feeling dizzy, asked to sit down. I sensed that this was as far as he could go, particularly with cigarettes and alcohol so much a part of his

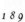

coping mechanism. I give him a hug, wrapping myself around his tall, lanky frame. He told me that the hugs might be the best part of the treatment. I agreed.

MOVING FROM THE MUSCLES

A writer I knew, learning of my interest in ALS, asked me if I would like to work with a remarkable woman with whom he had once studied acting. After I agreed, another acting student of Helene's called to arrange the appointment for her. The student, Jeannette, also told me what an extraordinary person Helene was, and how tragic the loss, particularly of the muscles that control speech, was for her. She also told me that a Reiki group had been treating Helene on a regular basis. I gathered that Helene had helped many others and, like all great teachers, had a grateful and devoted following.

Helene's apartment overlooking the East River was bright, cheerful, and filled with many objects of healing and devotion. Jeannette was also there, and I liked both women immediately. I felt from Helene, as I hugged her, love, trust, and sadness. She was losing strength in her hands, she told me; she couldn't easily hold her fingers apart and no longer had the strength to press the elevator bell to summon the machine to her floor.

Copying what Bonnie had shown me, I held one of her hands and put my other hand higher up on her arm, where there was no muscle weakness yet. Then I allowed my awareness to come down below the level of the repair cells in her muscles, to where I could feel a strong, equal pulse of energy in both places. I invited Jeannette to hold Helene's other hand and come energetically to the same place with me. This seemed easy for Jeanette, perhaps because of her experience with Reiki. "Helene, I'm below the level of the repair cells in your muscles," I told her. "I want you to allow your nerves to feel this energy and start spreading the pattern to other cells." Helene closed her eyes and seemed to drink in the force of this energy, which she said she felt in her whole body.

"Now I want you to practice moving your wrist from the muscles themselves, not through messages brought by the nerves," I told her. "First, just try flexing the wrist as you would normally do." She made a very weak movement of her wrist. "I'm going to show you the difference now between moving from the nerves and moving from the muscles." I held her forearm and her hand and flexed the wrist, without thinking about how I was doing it. "That's from the nerves," I told her. "Now we're going to do it from the muscles." I allowed my awareness to come into my own muscles and moved my hand, which was holding hers, from an impulse that came from the muscle alone. "I know it's slower," I said, "but can you feel the energetic difference as well?"

Helene nodded. "Good. Now I want you to do it, with me holding you." The first time she tried it, I found that I was doing all the work. "You're still not in your muscles," I said. "Let me show you again." This time she sank more into herself and flexed the wrist slowly but effortlessly within my grasp. To her delight, she found that using this method she could separate her fingers and bring them together again easily and press down very hard with any of them.

I then took out one of the ridged rubber balls and asked her to do the same exercise with her foot. As she did so, she began to cry. Her face was transformed into a mask of grief, her mouth opened, and sobs came from her throat. Something about the movement of the muscles in the foot had evoked an old and buried pain. I got the sense that some loving connection had been lost in her life. After the session she told me that she would be gone for a couple of weeks—that she was going south to visit her family, including her brother, who had been a very successful electrician but was now severely depressed and rarely left his house.

The next time I saw Helene, after she came back from her

trip, she told me that while she was practicing the movements with both her hand and her foot, she had meditated and gone inside her muscles to the repair cells, where I had told her the problem might have started. "I found a little man there, in total despair, sitting with his head between his hands," she said. "I knew it was my brother, Bob. I told him that he had to stop moping and to get up because he had work to do," Helene said. "His work was to repair my muscles."

How perfect, I thought, *and how much more suitable than anything I could have imagined.* "That makes sense," I said, "since it's the electric impulses in the nerves penetrating the muscles that have to do the work of healing. It feels to me as if you've held in your body a memory of your brother's competence—in fact, of his genius—which he has put aside or forgotten. I think that waking it up and using it in this way will be healing for both of you."

ATTENTION DEFICIT DISORDER

My next experience with what is generally thought of as a nervous system disorder was with Charlie, a bright, attractive teenager who was the son of a friend. I met him while I was visiting his mother and stepfather. Alvin, Charlie's stepfather, had a great interest in healing, and from time to time we had talked about the possibility of doing a television show or a series on the subject.

The conversation turned to my work, and I launched into one of my usual tirades about the crudeness of much of Western medical treatment. I described an article I had recently read that compared the mechanism of most pharmaceutical drugs to "hitting a fly with a sledgehammer." Although the purpose of a drug treatment might be to block only one receptor on the surface of a cell, the author explained, the chemical substances it contained were so powerful and generalized compared with the body's own exquisitely subtle and specific chemistry that it knocked out a hundred receptors instead of just one. Hence the noxious side effects.

"Besides," I said, "it doesn't deal with the issue of why that particular receptor has become overactive or oversensitive to begin with. It just temporarily knocks out the symptom, short-circuiting the feeling, which, although it may be expressed inappropriately, still needs to be addressed."

"You mean the drug could actually be harming you, by not letting you be who you really are?" Charlie, who was sitting next to me, suddenly piped up.

"Yes, in a manner of speaking," I said. Charlie gave his mother, Judith, a penetrating "I told you so" look.

Alvin explained, "Charlie was diagnosed with attention deficit disorder. He's been on Ritalin, and while it does allow him to concentrate on his schoolwork, he's not happy with the way it makes him feel."

"I'm very isolated," Charlie said. "I don't feel like going out or doing anything with my friends. Sure, I get my work done. That's because I'm home all the time." I felt a tug in my chest, and my usual arrogant conviction that there must be a better way rose up inside me. "Have you ever worked with anybody like me?" he asked, as if reading my thoughts.

"No," I said, "but I'd be glad to try."

"What would you do?" he asked.

"Well, I'd try to take you back to some time in your life when focusing was easier for you, and to see what was going on with your nervous system and your muscles then. I'd try to see what interrupted the ease and comfort of their coordination, making focused action so difficult for you." Alvin and Judith, clearly sensitive to Charlie's unhappiness, seemed enthusiastic about this approach. "All I'd ask you to do is not take the drug the day before you see me, and the day that you come."

A couple of weeks later, Judith and Charlie arrived at my house. Judith's love, concern, and anxiety for him, her only child, were obvious. She told me that she too had tremendous trouble concentrating at times and thought that she would have been diagnosed as ADD if that label had existed when she was a child.

As I talked to Judith, Charlie was clutching a cardboard tube filled with potato chips like a security blanket and eating them steadily. Judith was a superb gourmet cook, but Charlie for the most part disdained her cuisine, and food was an important issue between them. I mentioned to Charlie as gently as I could that diet might be a contributing factor to his problem, and that there was some evidence linking a high-fat, high-sugar, high-additive diet to hyperactivity. Judith reminded him that he had been on a restrictive diet for a while and it had seemed to work.

Since cravings for certain foods are strongly linked to emotional needs, I didn't want to push the point. Sugar and fat in particular bring back memories of mother's milk, which is high in both. "Maybe after we do some work together to support you energetically, you'll find it easier to go back on that healthier diet" was all I said.

We decided that it would be better for me to work with Charlie without Judith's being there (although in my practice now my preference is almost always to work with parents and children together), so she went to her car to spend the next hour reading. Charlie was attractive and engaging, obviously very bright, and a poignant sadness showed through his adolescent mantle of invulnerability. I started by suggesting that he get down on the floor and do some crawling. As he did so, the sense of sadness increased but no clear images came through. Then I had him lie on his back with his limbs stretched out and slowly contract his arms, legs, head, and hips, moving them all up and in toward his navel, like a starfish with six limbs, folding them all in to its center. He did this a few times. I told him to feel the energy moving in toward his navel as he contracted, then out from his navel to his extremities as he relaxed and expanded. I explained that on an energetic level this movement recapitulated the sensation of blood and energy flowing from his body through the umbilical cord, into his mother's body when he was inside her, and from her body back into his.

The sadness seemed to intensify as he continued, but again no images or powerful sweeps of feeling or energy came to me. Finally I had him lie on the couch, and I told him that I was going to take him even more powerfully, through his breathing, back to the experience of being inside the womb.

"First I want you to close your eyes and allow yourself to feel very light, as if you were floating down through the couch," I said, with my hands resting lightly on his feet. "I want you to feel as if you were made out of clouds, and the couch was made out of clouds. . . . Now I want you just to become aware of your breathing. Just notice the breath going in and out of your body. And notice also that the wonderful thing about breathing is that all you really have to do to make it work is to exhale— to let the air out of your body. As soon as you finish doing this, the universe sends the next breath rushing back into you. It is the universe's promise of support. All you really have to do is just let go."

I watched and felt Charlie relaxing more and more as I spoke, and I felt myself traveling to that relaxed and open place with him, carried there by our connection of trust. I allowed him to take several breaths in silence, and then I continued: "Now I want you to try a different kind of breathing. I want you to breathe as if you were breathing through your navel—as if you were drawing breath into your body at that central place—as if one great lung, just behind the navel, were drawing the air into your body." I saw his lower abdomen rise and fall in a gentle, even rhythm. "I want you to know, as you breathe in this way, through the navel, that this was how you breathed when you were inside your mother's body, and all oxygen and all nourishment came into you from her through your navel. This was how you breathed when your mother was breathing for you.

"Now I want you to feel yourself, there in your mother's womb, traveling back in time to the moment, sometime in the third month after conception, when all the neurons in your body that were designed to connect with muscle cells made those connections. Until now there has been no brain-directed movement in your body. You could not order a limb to move. But now feel each nerve cell finding its muscle cell—feel every muscle cell signaling and attracting the nerve that will be its partner for the rest of its life. I want you to feel that connection, those millions of connections, all over your body, being made. Now that the connections are made, I want you to make the first movement you feel impelled to make—your first brain-directed movement."

Charlie's left foot shot out, then drew back again as a bolt of fear ran through his body. I immediately got that it was his fear of hurting his mother—his sense that his focused action was a threat to her and something from which he must protect her. "Charlie, did you notice the fear that went through your body when you moved your foot?" I asked. He nodded without opening his eyes. "I think this is the key to your ADD," I said. "I think you got the message very early on that your focused action, independent of your mother but inside her, was some kind of threat to her. And so you made a decision that you wouldn't focus, that you would keep fragmenting your attention. I think you need to give yourself permission to focus now. Know that any fear that comes up comes from this very early time. Nothing bad is going to happen to you or your mother because of it now."

I said all this without wondering if it was more than a fourteen-year-old could absorb or understand. I remembered myself at fourteen, and my hunger for clues to my own distress. Something about Charlie's precocious intelligence reminded me of myself. "Why don't you open your eyes, sit up, and tell me how you're feeling?" I said. As he moved into a sitting position, the sadness seemed gone, and I was rewarded for my efforts with a wonderful open smile.

"My head feels light and clear," he said, "but it was weird."

"What was weird?" I asked, hoping for some gripping memory of prenatal life.

"It's weird to lie down when you're not sick and you're not going to sleep," he said.

"Oh, well, yes, I guess it is," I said, realizing that most adolescents, even in these sophisticated times, have not spent hour after hour on an analyst's couch.

When Charlie came back to see me two weeks later, he told me that he had not gone back to taking Ritalin and that he felt fine. I did a standard energy chelation on him, which he seemed to enjoy, but the major part of our work together was over for the time being. His issues were so intertwined with those of his mother that working with them both, either together or separately, would be the next step, but Judith didn't seem ready for that.

I don't know what instinct led me to take him back into his prenatal life, let alone that moment of nerve-to-muscle connection. In the literature I had read about the neurotrophic factor in the ALS trial, some mention had been made of its importance in attracting nerve cells to muscle cells in utero, and that had brought my attention to this prenatal event. I was forced to conclude, however, that some signal from Charlie himself had guided me back to that specific moment.

I later learned that Judith's first husband, Charlie's father, had been involved in some way with the Mafia and was murdered when Charlie was two, and that there had often been men with guns in the house when she was pregnant with him. When I saw him, Charlie knew nothing of the violence in which his parents had lived; he had been told that his father was killed by a burglar. Clearly, however, he had sensed the atmosphere of terror from inside his mother's body.

Although ADD ceased to be a problem, he continued to have a troubled life as an adolescent and was a long time coming to a secure and comfortable sense of himself.

Charlie's was but the first of my many journeys to the world of prenatal life, that supposedly unremembered time and place. I did not foresee that my approach to healing in general and surgery in particular would be subtly and powerfully changed by these voyages.

INFANT MEMORIES

Soon after I saw Charlie, I got a call from a woman who was in an obvious state of distress. One of the twin boys to whom Gladys had given birth almost a year earlier was born with a serious heart defect: only two instead of the normal four chambers had been formed. The proposed remedy was a series of operations, one of which had already been performed. Having had some experience of alternative therapies herself (she used both homeopathic remedies and Reiki during the pregnancy), she was calling me, she said, in a desperate attempt to avoid the future surgeries.

I had to tell Gladys in all honesty, given the seriousness of the condition she had described, that avoiding the surgeries might be impossible. I had never worked with an infant before, I told her, but I was confident that we could gain some insights into the baby's experience of his own heart, which could be helpful in any future treatment.

When Gladys and her son Steven arrived at my house, the first question that crossed my mind was what aspect of herself he represented to his mother. Presumably because his heart was not getting all the oxygen needed to all the cells in his body, she told me, Steven was lagging behind his twin brother developmentally. He could not hold his head up as easily, and his voice seemed stuck at a higher pitch. His care and healing had become her complete obsession. She also felt quite a bit of guilt about "abandoning" his brother on the night of the birth to go find Steven in the neonatal ICU, where she had become hysterical watching them "poke and prod at him."

Something moved me to ask her about the third month of gestation. "I was in Tortola," she said, "and not in very good shape. The winds kept howling and howling, and I think the bottled water I was drinking had come right out of the hotel tap."

"I have a feeling that something happened to Steven at that point," I said. I suggested that she hold him in her arms, which she did. He immediately nodded off to sleep. I put my hand over his tiny heart and told her that even though it might be uncomfortable for her, she should close her eyes and go back to that time in Tortola. As soon as she did so, I got an image of an older woman standing at a kitchen table, her head bowed in what seemed to be a state of despondency. "Gladys, was your mother depressed?" I asked.

"She was very depressed. She acted as if her whole life, and we children in particular, were some unbearable burden to her."

"I think Steven is carrying the feeling of her depression in his heart," I said. Tears started to roll down Gladys's cheeks from under her closed lids. "I also think that this feeling came into him, or he assumed responsibility for it, in the third month of gestation. I'm going to suggest that he release it. Steven," I said softly, "I want you to give back to your grandmother any of her sorrow that you absorbed through your mother. I want you to release it from your heart." As if on cue, Steven opened his eyes, smiling.

"Gladys," I said, trying to think of a way not to add to her already substantial guilt, "I think this is about your own need to separate from your mother, and that Steven somehow represents the part of you that hasn't done that yet. The most important thing you can really do for him is to focus on your own healing." To my relief, she seemed to accept this without resentment. She then told me that her husband was sometimes impatient with her ministrations to Steven, which I then saw as an attempt to take care of herself. I wondered to what extent both of them used the child and his illness as a way of avoiding dealing with other issues between them.

Later I learned that women very often unconsciously relive their own gestation when they are pregnant. Possibly when Gladys's mother was in the third month of her pregnancy with Gladys, this despair had overwhelmed her, and then Gladys had reexperienced it in her own third month with Steven.

A couple of days later, Gladys called me very excitedly to tell me that when she got Steven home, he was able to hold his head up with ease, and that his voice had gotten lower in its register and stronger. A couple of weeks later she brought him back for another session, and I did as much energy work on him as he would allow, running energy from each limb through the navel to the opposite limb, running it from one arm to the other, crossing the heart, and from the left arm to the head, and then to the base of the spine, connecting the heart with the brain and the genitals.

As with Charlie, however, I felt that the main piece of my work with him alone was finished, and that the work his mother did on herself would be critical for both their healing. Dr. Oz once told me, "I loved pediatric surgery, but the problem with it was that you always had two patients—the child and the mother." My work with both Steven and Charlie brought that truth home to me, along with the further, more complex issue that a child often expresses in his illness a whole family's pain or dysfunction.

Working with Infants

About the same time that I worked with Charlie, I got a call from a favorite professor of mine at the School of Public

Health. He was going in for knee surgery and wanted to know if I would be willing to prepare him for it and work with him in the OR. I was delighted—both because I respected and adored Dr. Challenor, whose concern for his students was always winningly evident, and because I had never worked in orthopedic surgery or with a patient under local anesthesia before.

For his part he had tried unsuccessfully to whip up some enthusiasm on the part of his surgeon for my being there during the operation. I got the definite sense that my presence was only grudgingly tolerated, since the surgeon neither addressed me nor made eye contact with me during the entire operation. Before the actual work of cutting the bone was begun, a technician from radiology came into the OR and gave us all aprons with lead shielding to wear. Then he wheeled the X-ray machine into place, and the bones of Dr. Challenor's knee appeared on the screen. The surgery itself was noisy work, done with tools that looked as if they belonged in a carpenter's or a stonemason's shop. I concentrated on keeping blood loss down by instructing Dr. Challenor, as I had forgotten to do in the prep, to let it pool in the other three limbs. Early on I got an image of a little boy running and then falling, with no one around to comfort him.

In contrast to the surgeon, the anesthesiologist was friendly and talkative. He told me that it was he who originated the practice of doing such surgeries under local rather than general anesthesia at Columbia, and that he'd like to bring some alternative methods of pain management into the hospital. He had a friend, a fellow South African, he said, who had taken a year off to study alternative medicine in London before taking a position as a neonatologist at the Hershey Medical Center at Penn State.

Within the week I was on the phone to Charles Palmer at Penn State, who asked me to fax him anything I had written describing my work. When we spoke again, he said, "I have two questions for you: Can I learn to do what you do, and would it work with infants?" I told him that the answer to both was yes.

I spent a couple of days at Hershey, taking stock of the situation in the neonatal ICU and meeting with a group of people who shared Charles's interest in alternative medicine. At the group meeting someone asked for a demonstration—a request that always sends a bolt of fear running through me when I'm not prepared for it. A medical anthropologist volunteered to be the subject, and I decided, partly to prevent boredom, to involve everyone in the room in the process. I stood with my hands on the subject's head and asked the others to position themselves so they could touch his hands, feet, and abdomen. Everyone said that they could feel the energy moving through his body as I worked and as he went into a very deep state of trance. Moving down to put my hand on his chest, I felt ancient sorrow connected with his father and more recent sorrow with his son, who I later discovered had some serious psychological problems. Without naming this issue, I suggested that he release into my hand and the safe space we were creating around him whatever he was holding in his chest. He got off the conference table feeling slightly dizzy and disoriented but lighter and easier in his body and convinced of the power of this process.

Later, Charles took me into the neonatal ICU, where babies, many of them premature, struggled for life in cribs and "isolettes." I stepped up to one and tuned in with Charles standing next to me. *Terror, fourth month,* a voice inside my brain told me as I watched the tiny chest straining to take in air. "Whatever was going on with this infant started in the fourth month of gestation," I told Charles. "And she's still feeling the fear of it." We stepped over to another one, and a feeling of abandonment and despair swept through me. "I think her mother went into despair around the sixth month, and she felt as if her mother were leaving her," I said to Charles. "I think you could do important healing for both of them, if the mother could acknowledge this and hold her, or at least touch the isolette, as she talks about what happened to her during the pregnancy."

When we got to the next crib, I told him that an image of

a very angry father was coming to me. "I don't know if it's just the power of suggestion, Julie," Charles said, "but I'm starting to pick up the same messages that you're getting."

"Anyone who cares as much as you do could pick them up," I said. "What it takes is that feeling of caring, and then being with someone who does it, so that you can tune your consciousness to the same place and give yourself permission to take the signals you're getting seriously."

Charles was concerned both with measuring the effectiveness of the work and with finding a way to describe it to his fellow physicians in a way that would allow them to both understand it and accept it. He came up with the wonderful idea of presenting what I did as an extension of a normal medical examination. "In other words, Julie," he said, "you'll be offering them another tool for their kit bag. You'll be teaching them how to observe and record additional relevant data, albeit of a somewhat different kind, about their patients."

"Yes," I said excitedly, "and as people who consider themselves scientists, they have to understand the value of having all this additional data." This notion was, of course, a little naive on my part. The importance of a person's emotional history to his physical well-being has long been acknowledged in medical circles, but once that person passes through the doors of a medical institution, it is largely ignored. The mystery is why this continues to happen. What is the investment in continuing to act, against all evidence, as if feelings have so little impact on the internal actions of the body?

Of course, it is not just doctors who experience schizophrenia around this information. If patients were not coconspirators, the distortion would not continue.

My work with my next patient brought into focus an important insight about the meaning of hospitalization in general and surgery in particular.

The woman at the other end of the telephone line, Violet, introduced herself as a psychotherapist struggling with heart problems and a possible diagnosis of breast cancer. She was not being treated well by her physicians, she felt, but she was afraid of angering them by challenging their sometimes dismissive responses to her questions and concerns. Later, sitting in the living room of her apartment filled with beautiful examples of African art, I listened to her expanding on this theme, as her eyes darted nervously all around the room. I was reminded of how strongly people recreate parental relationships with their doctors.

She was unhappy, she told me, with her short, squat body, but she couldn't give up the comfort of the foods that filled in so much of her loneliness. She was also angry at her body for betraying her through disease. She did, however, find release and pleasure in two very physical activities: dance therapy and painting. When she danced, she told me, a freedom and lightness came into her body, and she experienced love for herself and a connection to the rest of the universe. The painting satisfied her need to express what she felt inside in some external form.

As Violet talked about these creative and healing outlets, her face relaxed, and I was impressed once again with people's ability to seek out and find what they need to nurture themselves. Part of our work together, I told her, would be to find out what was keeping her from having the feeling about her body that dancing brought her all the time, and to release it if we could.

In her office she lay down on a couch, and I was drawn to put my hands over her distended lower abdomen. I got an image of a very forlorn-looking little girl, and when I told her about it, she told me about her feeling of being ignored by her narcissistic mother. Under the sorrow that was now welling up in her, I felt the explosive force of her anger. When I suggested she get up and do an anger exercise, however, she declined, saying it might upset the neighbors. A defensive part of me leaped up at that point and wanted to challenge her. "How can you call yourself a therapist when you have your office someplace where people can't even yell?" my Miss Know-It-All would have liked to say. But I caught this intolerant little tyrant, always ready to dictate rules of health and healing to others, and put her back in her box. A wiser, less easily threatened part of myself understood that people came to Violet for the healing she could give them, which was the healing they were ready for and needed at that moment in their lives.

When the session was over, Violet said that she would like to work with me again. During the next session I asked her to reach energetically, beyond her mother, to a connection with her father, and to feel him holding her hand. I took her hand in mine as I did so. "Feel his love coming down into your body as he holds your little hand in his," I said. Her breathing deepened, and a sense of profound relaxation took over her body. Tears rolled down her cheeks.

About a week later she called to tell me that a biopsy had revealed the need for a lumpectomy, which she would have done by a surgeon at Mount Sinai. I told her that I'd be glad to work with her before, during, and after the surgery, and that because of my grant from the Symington Foundation, there would be no charge to her for the work. She seemed hesitant when I told her that I had not worked with this surgeon before, nor gone into the OR at this hospital, and that she would have to ask him for permission. "I'll think about it," she said.

When she called me back, I could tell by the way she inhaled before speaking that she was not going to go for it. "I don't want to upset him by asking for anything extra," she said. Knowing that it was not an emergency surgery, I asked if she would consider going to a surgeon at another hospital with whom I'd worked before. "No, no. This surgeon is a friend of my cardiologist's, and I don't want to make him angry." I tried to explain that patients switch surgeons and hospitals all the time and for all kinds of reasons, but to no avail. She asked if she could hire me just to do the pre- and post-op work, and I said of course.

We met again about a week before her surgery. She lay down on the couch, and I put my hands lightly on either side of her head. "Violet, I want you to imagine that you are lying on a gurney in the hospital, and very loving hands are pushing you very gently through the corridor—"

"Those aren't loving hands," she snapped. "I've been to that hospital. Those people are brutal, the way they push you around."

"All right," I said with a sigh. "Then I want you to imagine yourself lying on the operating table. And as the anesthesiologist very carefully puts the needle into your arm, I want you to—"

"They're not careful," she said. "They're all in a hurry, and they're completely indifferent to what I feel."

"Violet," I said, my heart sinking, but knowing better than to contradict her, "maybe you shouldn't be having this surgery now. Maybe you should put it off, or think again about having it done somewhere else."

"I don't want to hear that from you!" she said, almost screaming.

"Fine," I said. "Whatever feels comfortable for you. But I don't think this kind of preparation is going to help you right now. Why don't I just do some energy work and relax you as much as possible?" She agreed, and I worked almost in silence, directing energy to the breast that would be operated on, to her lymphatic system, and to her heart. She thanked me at the end of the session, and I told her that I would be out of town at a conference the following week but would call her when I got back.

When I returned home two days after Violet's surgery, I called the hospital and asked for her. I was told that she was in the cardiac critical care unit. One of the nurses on duty told me that Violet had crashed (gone into cardiac arrest) on the operating table and was in the unit with pulmonary edema (lungs filled with fluid). My own lungs seemed to cave in as I heard the news. One surgeon whom I'd worked with, I remembered, had told me that no one in his right mind would operate on a patient who didn't think he was going to survive the surgery.

When I went to see Violet the next day, I was struck as I entered the lobby by the forbidding nature of the hospital's architecture, which seems reminiscent of a high-tech jail. Inside the unit, however, there were large, airy individual rooms with windows for each patient, in contrast to the dark, dreary cubicles at Columbia. Violet was intubated with her hands strapped to the sides of the bed—to keep her from pulling out the breathing tube and the intravenous lines, the nurse explained. She was also hooked up to monitors that read out her vital signs, like heart rate and blood pressure. There was a wild, frightened look in her eyes, but she did hold my gaze when I stepped in front of the bed, and she seemed glad to see me. "I'm so sorry that this happened," I said.

I put my hands lightly on her feet, and her eyes closed. I moved my thumbs to the kidney point at the bottom of each foot. The throb of energy was faint, but gradually it strengthened under my touch. Since the kidneys are a key factor in controlling the balance of liquids in the body, I hoped that this would help her drowning lungs. I put my hands directly over her lungs and stimulated the lung meridians by touching points on the outside of the nails on her thumbs and a couple of inches down from the center of her collarbone on each side. When I had finished, I noticed that both her pulse and her blood pressure had come down to almost normal levels.

One of the nurses came into the room, followed by the intern on duty. Neither of them either looked at or talked to Violet. Instead, they went over to one of the monitors and started discussing "the case" as if she weren't in the room. I looked over at Violet, who was now looking over at them, and saw in her eyes a longing for recognition and contact. I wanted to beg the intern to at least say hello to her patient, but since I was there at the sufferance of the medical staff, such a request would be considered, at the very least, inappropriate. As they were talking, Violet's heart rate and blood pressure shot up again. After they left, I told her that I too had to leave, but that I would be back in a day or two. As I leaned over the railing of the bed, maneuvering around all the devices attached to her, for a hug, I realized that hospital beds, with their raised sides, are like cribs. And patients in critical and intensive care units like Violet, strapped down and helpless, intubated so they cannot speak, are like infants, completely dependent upon people to whom they cannot communicate their needs and desires.

It occurred to me then that much about staying in a hospital recapitulated all the worst aspects of a childhood in which your physical needs were minimally taken care of and your emotional needs completely ignored. I began to think that people came to hospitals to reenact their childhoods, and that it was usually just as bad the second time around. What a difference it would make, though, if patients could acknowledge their need for loving parenting, and if physicians and other health care providers could embrace this as part of their job description.

Healing in the Workplace

I had always considered myself a diehard northeasterner, devoted to the intellectual vortex that spirals around New York City. Anyone I ever wanted to meet in any field of activity, it seemed, sooner or later passes through that throbbing mesh of stone, steel, money, and brains at the mouth of the Hudson River.

During a trip to San Francisco to take a workshop, however, I found myself captivated by the Bay Area and its more open attitude about healers and healing. Judith Tolson, associate director of the Institute for Health and Healing at California Pacific Medical Center, suggested that I come out the following year as a visiting professor, giving grand rounds in medicine and psychiatry, a public lecture, and a workshop. The prospect of missing a wet, cold, snowy winter in the Northeast loomed appealingly before me, and I applied for a grant from the Susan G. Komen Foundation (the largest private funders of breast cancer research in the country) to continue my work in breast cancer surgery in the Bay Area.

On this first trip for the workshop, I got a call from a friend of someone I'd treated in New York. Tamara was a fashion designer and a breast cancer survivor who had had a bizarre accident: an imperfectly shelled shrimp had stuck in her throat and scratched it badly. Since then she'd had persistent pain and discomfort in her throat, for reasons the doctors couldn't explain.

When I met Tamara in her studio, I put my hands on her throat and immediately got a feeling of rage vibrating between my palms. I suggested to Tamara that there was something she needed to yell about. "I think it's about your mother," I said, the words coming out of my mouth before I could think. We ended up at a deserted place on the waterfront, where Tamara connected very quickly to the feeling. Her voice slammed like a machine gun into the tree on whose trunk I had told her to visualize her mother. When the feeling crested, when the word "liar" seemed to fly out of her without effort, her center of gravity lowered, as if she herself were becoming planted in the ground. As we drove back to her office, she told me that she'd like to get a group of people together to experience my work.

A couple of days later I went back to the studio, where a small group of Tamara's employees and friends were assembled. I talked a little bit about tuning in to people's energy to read and rebalance the emotions blocked in their bodies. Some kind of group healing seemed the most effective way to let them all experience what I was talking about, and Tamara suggested that the subject be her bookkeeper, who was having trouble walking after a skiing accident and had become very depressed about it.

I had the bookkeeper, Anna, lie down on a long work table, and I positioned the other people around her, touching her hands, feet, arms, and legs, while I stood at her head. I instructed the people to maintain eye contact with each other across her body as we worked so that energy would be exchanged both through her and across her. "What was happening when the accident occurred?" I asked.

"Nothing," she said. "It was a beautiful day, and I was out with some friends skiing."

"Can you remember what you were thinking about, just before you fell?" I asked.

"They were up ahead of me, and I was worrying if I was going to be able to catch up with them, or if they would leave me behind. They were very good skiers." A slight catch came into her throat as she said this, and her voice got higher, like a little girl's.

"It's a terrible feeling to be left behind," I said. "I want you to take a deep breath, Anna, and say as you exhale, 'Come back here!'"

"Come back here," she said very softly.

"Let yourself say it in a high, little girl's voice," I instructed.

"Come back here!" she called. "Come back here!" Fear and finally anger were in her voice.

"Let them know you mean it," I said. She began to sob and then became very quiet and calm. Everyone touching her had also gone to that deep and quiet place. "I want you to take in from each of us touching you now exactly what you need that we have to offer. And know that taking it is the greatest gift you can give us." We stayed like that for a few minutes. Two of the other employees were crying.

"You know, I work with these people all the time," Tamara

told me when we had finished, "but we almost never touch each other."

"And you almost never have the experience of just looking into someone's eyes for more than a moment," a friend of hers said. "It's so—so intimate."

"Yes, the eyes have energy," I said. "They both give off and receive light."

Tamara thanked me for healing her throat, which had felt relaxed, open, and pain-free since we worked, and for healing her bookkeeper's leg and spirits. I began to get a sense of what work could really be like in this country if people looked upon their workplaces as places of healing as well as production. If they began the workday by doing very simple energetic connections like looking and touching. If once a day or even once a week, for just twenty minutes, people came together to focus healing energy on someone with whom they worked.

People recreate their family relationships and power structures at work all the time, I thought, probably in some hope of healing them through parallel action. Since they do so unconsciously, however, they usually create situations where they don't feel any safer about defending themselves than they did at home as children, and they end up rewounding themselves. Making healing a conscious part of working would acknowledge these recreations of family interactions and offer freedom from them. It would also free up a great deal of energy for productivity.

Chapter Eleven

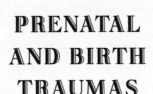

PRENATAL AND BIRTH TRAUMAS

After my experience in the CCU with Violet, I had found myself wondering, if people go into critical care units to become infants, what do they go into the operating room for? Then it hit me: to go back to the womb. The moment the thought came to me, the pieces flew together. Under general anesthesia, you hear but you don't see. Some outside source breathes for you (and, in the case of cardiac surgery, actually oxygenates and degasses your blood for you). With the muscle relaxant they use, the nerves fire but the muscles don't respond, as in the first three months after conception. Dramatic changes, often involving the transfer of tissue from one place to another, take place in your body. And unless you are later brought back there by hypnosis, you have complete amnesia of the event. When else but in gestation does any state like this happen?

Soon after I had this insight that surgery reactivates the trauma of gestation, I was called to work on a very unusual case. Carla, a woman in her forties, had a congenital condition that had just been discovered and diagnosed and was threatening to paralyze her and possibly end her life. She had been born with a longer-than-normal odontoid bone (the bone at the top of the spinal column). Although the condition had caused her no trouble for most of her life, the bone was now pressing on her brain stem. If she turned her head to the right, everything looked askew. She was nauseated every day.

The proposed remedy involved two operations, performed two days apart. During the first surgery the surgeon would enter her mouth, make an incision at the back of her throat, and drill through to remove a piece of the bone. Two days later he would go in through the back of her neck and fuse the occiput and first and second cervical vertebrae. It was a relatively new procedure that had been done fewer than twenty times in New York, all of them by Dr. De Los Reyes at Beth Israel North. There was a possibility that Carla would emerge from the surgery with complete and irreversible paralysis. But there was also a chance, if all went well, that after a few months of rest and immobilization, she would go back to living a relatively normal, healthy, and active life. She had been warned, however, that she would always be in some degree of pain and have limited mobility in her neck.

Carla had heard about my work from a colleague who had seen me on television, and she told me that she was hiring me to give herself "every chance she could possibly have." I met her at her office, and we did a session on the carpeted floor of a nearby room to prepare her for the first surgery. She had endured an unhappy first marriage, she told me, one that she had entered into in order to escape from an unhappy family situation. Now, however, she was married to a man who treasured her and with whom she was experiencing, in her own words, happiness beyond anything she ever had dreamed possible. Her joy showed clearly in her face.

I started by working at Carla's feet, pulling on her big toes to release some of the tension in her neck and head. Then I put

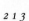

my hands on her head, which I would be holding during the first surgery, and led her through what would be happening to her, step by step. She thanked me for the session, saying she felt very calm and confident about the surgery, and very relaxed as a result of the healing.

The following week, an hour before the surgery was scheduled to begin, I met Carla and her husband at the hospital. The anesthesiologist gave her Valium beforehand, but as she was wheeled into the OR, a panicked feeling of kicking and screaming was in her body. A feeling of choking was in her throat when the area to be operated on was X-rayed.

The throat represents the umbilical cord, the place through which air and nourishment pass into the body. The first and second cervical vertebrae are where memories are held of the time when the embryo grows out from the uterine wall into the space of the uterus itself. This first act of individuation and separation from the mother comes just after conception, when the mother first misses her period and suspects that she might be pregnant.

As Carla went under anesthesia, there was a sense of both hysteria and pain, strongly focused in her uterus. Then her entire being seemed to sink into profound despair. As Dr. De Los Reyes drilled into the bone, there was a sense of chaos, then dizziness. I got a picture of a little girl in terror and then in a terrible rage. When the first piece of bone was cut, relief swept through Carla's body, and when the odontoid was completely removed, there was an ecstatic feeling, followed by nausea.

I was so fascinated by the surgery that I forgot my intention of telling Carla to consciously focus on her life in the womb. Dr. De Los Reyes asked me if the energy in the room usually shifts when something starts to go wrong in a surgery. "Yes, it usually does," I said.

"Would you tell me if you notice anything like that?" he asked. He clearly had no embarrassment about his interest in my work, and I felt myself being treated with more respect than I ever had before. Fortunately there were no such energy shifts. Instead, a wonderful feeling of respect, affection, and cooperation between Dr. De Los Reyes, his physician's assistant, and the nurses gave the OR a sense of lightness. "When neurosurgery works," the PA told me, "it's the greatest thing in the world. But when it doesn't, there's nothing worse."

In the intensive care unit the next day, Carla was in extremely good spirits. I prepared her for the second surgery and told her this time that she might be going back to the womb, and that I would be there to help her process anything traumatic that came up.

During the second surgery, as she went under the anesthesia, I got an image of a fetus in terror. For the rest of the operation there was a deep but sweet pain feeling, as if love from every hand that touched her were flooding in to heal an ancient wound.

A few weeks after this surgery, Carla called me to tell me that she'd had much less pain than had been anticipated and was recovering way ahead of schedule. "The first time the physical therapist came to my house," she told me, "he had instructions just to roll me over in my bed so I wouldn't get bedsores. When I opened the door myself, fully dressed, he nearly fainted." In her long-term recovery she was virtually pain free and had almost complete mobility in her neck, despite predictions to the contrary.

My own hunch was that consciously processing prenatal trauma during the surgery was key to Carla's recovery, and I decided to make this a part of all my surgical work in the future.

LIFE BEFORE BIRTH

It was my observation of the role that the prenatal lives of my patients played in their experience of surgery that led to my interest in the work of William Emerson, a psychologist who had been working in the area of prenatal, birth, and neonatal trauma for over twenty years. Sometime after Carla's surgery, my friend Stephaine Mines, a jin shin jitsu practitioner and teacher, told me about William's work and her experience of it. Because of my insight that patients were traveling back to the womb during surgery, I was eager to learn everything I could about trauma in the first nine months of life, so I signed up for William's next workshop, scheduled in Boulder.

In the six weeks before the workshop I found myself in one of the worst depressions of my life. Nothing seemed to help. I was seeing a therapist with whom a lot of memories of a very troubled infancy came up, but each insight brought only temporary relief. The sun would pour through the clouds for twelve or twenty-four hours, only to have the gloom settle in again.

William's workshop catapulted me out of the depths of that depression as if it were shooting me out of a cannon. I thought I had come for my patients, but of course the most immediate and greatest beneficiary of this extraordinary experience was me. William introduced us to the idea that trauma experienced in the womb and during birth is held in specific places in the energy field around the body; that it could be felt in the field, reactivated through the field, and processed and released through loving observation, touch, energy, breathing, movement, and sound.

One of the coping mechanisms for dealing with this very early trauma, he said, is going into shock—sympathetic shock (a high-adrenaline state) for some people, and parasympathetic shock (a shot-down, lethargic state) for others. This shock is very easily triggered in later life, when memory of the trauma is close to the surface.

The original cause of the trauma may have been physical. For example, smoking on the part of the mother reduces the fetus's oxygen supply dramatically. Drinking and drug-taking send toxins into the tiny body that it is ill equipped to deal with. Or the cause can be emotional. If the child is not wanted or if there is hostility between the parents during the pregnancy, the tiny being trying to form itself knows it and is deeply affected by it. This communication comes both vibrationally (energetically) and chemically. Any stress hormones produced in the mother's body go directly from her bloodstream into that of the fetus, who has no way of filtering them out or distinguishing them from the hormones its own body is producing. If the mother or father suffers from depression during the pregnancy, it is communicated to the fetus. Very often one or both parents unconsciously reexperience the trauma of their own gestation during the pregnancy, and this is also passed on.

Birth trauma, William said, often recapitulates the trauma of those first nine months.

In the workshop we palpated the energy field around our partners to identify times of trauma in their prenatal and birth history. William also led us in group regressions, taking us back through conception, gestation, and birth.

I was astonished by the amount of information that came to me about those circumstances in my own life. At one point William worked on me to demonstrate some of his techniques to the group. Since my eyes were closed, I couldn't see what he was doing. All I knew was that he was holding his hand somewhere above my body and bringing his awareness to the time in my history that corresponded to the place in the energy field where traumatic memories were held. When his hand (as someone later told me) was over the crown of my head, I had a sensation of my father's fear at the moment of my conception. Family lore was that at the time when my parents had conceived me, they had been full of confidence that my father's new job, with a firm he had formed with friends, would make having a second child financially viable. At some point during the pregnancy, however, those friends betrayed him and threw him out of the company. My mother, who had never trusted them to begin with, became furious, then depressed.

As William wordlessly took me back to the sperm's awareness during the time of conception, it came to me that my father had either already lost the job or feared that he was going to lose it. But he wanted this child so badly that he decided not to tell my mother until the pregnancy was confirmed. Hence his fear at the very moment that he was creating me.

The other memorable experience I had as William worked on me was a feeling of being ignored because my parents were preoccupied with fighting with each other. This was certainly a constant memory from my earliest childhood, but I'd had no idea that it had depressed me so profoundly in the womb as well.

In the group regression William told us to imagine both the planet and our families in the year we were conceived. At first I was very excited by how beautiful the earth looked. Then I realized that it was 1942 and the Second World War was going on, and I felt frightened and sad. When I saw my parents and my three-year-old brother, an enormous resistance came up in me. "There must be some mistake," I said to the universe. "This is some kind of terrible joke. You can't possibly be sending me there. I don't want to go!" It was too late. I was already headed for incarnation, and there was no way to put on the brakes.

My birth, which I reenacted with a partner, felt exhausting. I barely had the energy to push my way through the birth canal, and I didn't seem to be getting any help at all from my mother. Part of her inaction, I'm certain, came from the fact that she was anesthetized—standard procedure in those days. But another part was that the very idea of being born seemed overwhelmingly depressing to me. Months later, when I did this exercise again, I sensed that even in her drugged state my mother withdrew from the sexuality of the experience and the excitement of that contact with me as I moved through her.

My grandmother had not wanted a fourth child, I knew, and had thought about having my mother aborted. I wondered now how my mother's unprocessed feelings about that had affected our entire relationship from the very beginning.

The workshop left me feeling transformed, with no hint of the depression that had weighed me down for the previous six weeks. I began to posit that perhaps deep and otherwise intractable areas of emotional distress, like clinical depression and addiction, have their roots in prenatal life.

In William's experience, he had said, memories of prediscovery trauma (before the pregnancy is confirmed) are held in the field around the sternum, while the discovery trauma itself (how parents react to the knowledge of the pregnancy) is held in the field around the sternal notch. This would mean that going for open heart surgery would strongly reactivate these traumas because the sternum, starting at the notch, is sawed in two. Are people who go in repeatedly for bypass surgery, I wondered, trying on an unconscious level over and over again to process this trauma?

William also said that there is an axis of energy that runs from the hollow between the collarbones, back through the neck to the first and second cervical vertebrae, which hold traumatic memories from the moment in gestation that represents the child's first act of individuation and separation from the mother. This is the time when the conceptus, which has attached itself to the uterine wall and been covered over by it, grows back out into the space of the womb, attached to the wall by a tiny stalk that eventually becomes the umbilical cord and the placenta. When he said this, I flashed back to an experience I'd had in my healing group a few weeks after Carla's surgery.

Four of us had been standing very close, hugging each other in a circle, in womblike coziness, when I wanted desperately to get away but felt embarrassed and a little crazy, since everyone was putting out such a loving feeling. Finally I just couldn't stand the tension anymore and pushed myself away, saying, "I've got to get out of here." My cousin Michael, who was standing next to me, put one hand on my back and the other on the top of my head. I immediately contracted my neck, jamming my head almost between my shoulder blades, and I said hysterically, "I know why people's upper vertebrae get fused." It came to me that it had something to do with my own experience in the womb, but I wasn't certain just what.

What I realized from William's identification of this vector was that Carla's surgery and my womblike experience had triggered a memory in me of my own prenatal trauma at that time. It was also the place where I had injured myself in the acrobatics accident so many years before, the event that had set me on the path of healing. Realizing all this, I was very eager to go back specifically to that point in my prenatal life, but time in the workshop just didn't allow for that.

My opportunity to do so came a couple of months later, when I was back in Boulder visiting Stephanie for Thanksgiving. I asked her if she would be willing to do some prenatal work with me, and she agreed, combining it with some jin shin jitsu in our sessions together. My first impulse was to go back to that time of growing out into the uterus. When we tried, starting with the moment of being inside the uterine wall, I got a headache that was so severe that we had to stop. We decided to reenact my birth instead, which this first act of separation would have prefigured. Trauma often has to be worked on in regressive layers, starting with a later manifestation before going back to the earliest instance.

The reenactment of my birth this time brought out that the exhaustion I'd experienced before was really a state of shock, triggered by my terror of coming into the family situation that I knew awaited me.

The next day we tried the prenatal work again, and this time I had no headache when I went back to being embedded in my mother's uterine wall. I said to Stephanie quite spontaneously, "I know everything about my mother."

"What do you mean?" she asked.

"I know the history of the Jews in Poland." What I saw in a flash was men on horseback shooting people. Specifically at that moment I knew the history of the Jews during my maternal grandmother's life there—the history of exclusion, oppression, and murder. I realized then that the dysfunction in my mother's family and in our own was an unconscious reflection of this history. A wave of compassion for my mother swept through me.

This insight immediately transformed all my thinking about the impact of culture on personality. In America, as a member of what was the dominant culture, I had never completely understood my black friends' deeply personal reactions to discrimination. In fact, I had often thought that if they would just focus on what their parents had done to them, they would be a lot better off. I even saw the focus on the abuses of the dominant society as a way of avoiding family issues. I now realized that there is no way to separate the violence within a family from the violence outside it—that each is a reenactment and a recapitulation of the other.

Next I did the part of the regression that involved growing out from the uterine wall into the space of the uterus itself. Terror seized me, and I found myself pulling my head down into my shoulders just as I had done that day in the group. I knew that this was the moment when I was in my mother but no longer completely of her. At that moment she identified me as something separate from herself, out of her control and therefore threatening.

Before this moment of individuation, I had had the feeling that I could heal my mother completely if I could just stay where I was, tucked inside the wall of her uterus, loving her in secret. I felt, however, that I desperately needed more oxygen, that not enough was coming into me, and that I had to keep growing to survive.

My experiences with memories of prenatal and birth trauma had a profound influence on my practice and on my understanding of both the disease process and treatment. I took four more workshops with William over the next six months and did extensive work on my own exploring these themes as well. I became interested in working with teenage parents and developing protocols that would allow them to reexperience their own gestation and birth before their child was born. Teenagers have babies, I became convinced, because they are trying desperately to reexperience their own troubled lives as infants and to heal them. If this process could be made conscious, I believe, multiple pregnancies might not occur.

Chapter Twelve

~~~~~

THE MANY
MEANINGS OF
SURGERY

The grant from the Komen Foundation came through, allow-ing me to work with twenty women having breast cancer surgery in the Bay Area. About the same time I got a grant from the Nathan Cummings Foundation to run an experimental en-ergy healing group for cardiac patients. My original plan had been to do the cardiac group at Beth Israel with Steve Horowitz's patients, but at the time that hospital's administration wanted to limit his involvement in alternative therapies, arguing that they were not bringing in as much money as operations like the catheterization laboratory. Accordingly, I decided to do the work with patients at California Pacific instead.

I arrived in San Francisco and almost immediately found myself surrounded by other healers. Most of them thought I could provide them with access to the medical world, especially to surgical patients. Many of them told me that they had had dreams or visions of working in surgery, or felt "pulled" in that direction. But my own entry into the field of healing in general and surgery in particular had had none of this sense of following a calling. In fact, all I seemed to be following each time I had taken another step was my own curiosity.

With perfect hindsight, however, I could see that secret engines had been pushing me: a certain unacknowledged competitiveness with my brother; an identification with people at war with bodies that bring them pain; and a desire to feel and witness over and over again the miracle of entering those bodies, when the residual effects of trauma made it difficult for me to consistently inhabit my own. My very disconnection from my own physical presence in the world, of which I was becoming more and more aware, made the extreme physicality of surgery compellingly attractive to me.

STANDING IN THE SURGEON'S SHOES

In this connection, I had a very interesting experience in San Francisco with a Russian healer of some renown. I saw him at the recommendation of a friend who had been studying with him. I had previously spoken with him about his theories of healing, which relate to a new concept of physics. But whether because of language difficulties or reticence, he hadn't been very forthcoming on that occasion, and so experiencing his work for myself seemed the best way to get an understanding of it.

Nikolai's technique was familiar to me because I had worked with other Russian healers. He waved his hands around my upper body, and very soon I found myself going into a trancelike state. What was unique in this experience was that I saw wavy lines in the air around me, which he later said were manifestations of the energy field he was creating. The next thing I knew, I felt myself standing in surgery: one of the surgeons I'd worked with at Columbia was to my right, as he usually was, working on a cardiac patient. Almost immediately after that I had the sensation that my hands were in his hands and that I was feeling what he felt inside the patient's body. Then I was completely in his body. A bolt of electric excitement went up my spine, as well as the thought *This person could die at any moment.* In that instant I realized that his excitement about cardiac surgery was exactly about this feeling of being on the edge of life and death.

When I related my experience to Nikolai, he looked very grave. I was entering the surgeon's body and taking in both his feeling and the feeling of the patient, he said, and this was dangerous for me. Detachment is the essence of effective healing, he told me, and without it I was injuring myself. For my own health, I had to stop working in surgery.

Of course I had no intention of doing any such thing. To begin with, I'd just accepted a grant to work in twenty surgeries. Even more important, I was in complete disagreement with his philosophy of healing. Not detachment but profound emotional involvement was at the very core of my work.

People often ask me what I do about the "bad energy" I take in from the people I do healing work with. I used to say simply that I don't take it in: I experience what they're feeling as a kind of ripple of energy passing through me and out again. Then a very clear explanation of this experience of "taking in," which some people doing healing work experience, was given to me by the singer Susan Osborne. "If an issue comes up for someone that you, as a healer, haven't dealt with in yourself," she said, "then it activates your own unresolved emotions, and you experience it as a 'bad feeling.' You haven't taken anything in from the other person. Your own stuff has gotten stimulated." This made perfect sense to me. It also made me wonder by what quirk of fate I seemed to attract only patients who were dealing with things I'd resolved in my life—albeit sometimes just the day before they showed up on my doorstep.

What interested me most about my session with Nikolai was that it made sense out of a psychic reading I'd had a few months before. Since I'd neglected to tell the psychic my two biases (no past lives and no alien abductions—I just don't believe in them), she came up with a vision of me, gowned, gloved, and male, working in an operating room, which she claimed was from a past life. She said I was up to my forearms in blood, and that I had been an obstetrical surgeon working in the nineteenth century on my wife, who died in childbirth. After my experience with Nikolai, I concluded that what she was actually picking up on was the fact that I had unconsciously been experiencing what cardiac surgeons were feeling when I worked with them, and the gestation and birth that their patients were reexperiencing during surgery.

THE BODY SPEAKS—AND WEEPS

There are many ways of reconstructing a breast, some of them using the body's own tissue, some of them using implants, and some using a combination of the two. Like so many other aspects of surgery, a woman's choice, not just about whether to reconstruct or not but about what kind of reconstruction to have, can be influenced by her emotional history.

The first breast cancer surgery case I did in San Francisco was with a strikingly attractive and sensual woman in her late thirties. Rebecca was scheduled for a re-op (redoing of an operation) for a reconstructive surgery she'd had at the time of her mastectomy. In her reconstruction, part of the latissimus dorsi muscle, from the back of her body, had been swung under her arm and, in combination with a saline implant, had been used to create a breast. Rebecca was displeased with the way the implant looked and the fact that it was too large. In addition, the wound on her back hadn't been healing properly and needed to be cleaned out. To complete her despair, the surgeon who had done the mastectomy had forgotten to leave the nipple on the body, as she'd been instructed to do. The surgeon, whom Rebecca trusted and liked, was so obviously distraught about this herself that Rebecca felt she couldn't be angry at her.

Reconstruction was essential for her, she told me, because her breasts had always been a part of her sense of her physical beauty, and showing off her body had been one of her delights. The scar on her back was especially troubling. She had always loved the look of her naked back and often wore dresses that displayed it.

Perhaps because Californians worship the body the way New Yorkers worship the mind, I encountered this kind of attitude toward the disfigurement of mastectomy much more frequently out there than I did in my breast cancer patients back east.

I put my hand on Rebecca's back over the scar and was immediately seized with a feeling of weeping. "Did anyone ever hit you when you were a child?" I asked.

"My father used to beat me—on my back," she said.

"I don't think we have to look any further for the reason that the wound hasn't healed. I think that you're still furious with him about it. There is no excuse to hit a child, and beating is outrageous. It's a terrible abuse of power."

I put my hands gently on her shoulders, which were extremely tense. Rebecca began to cry. "That feeling is rage," I said, "not pain. You can release some of that anger now, and then we can deal with whatever else comes up during the surgery. Why don't you stand up and face the wall?" She got up shakily and planted herself in front of a blank space of the wall, as I directed her to stand with her feet a shoulder's width apart and make fists. "I want you take a deep breath, and say 'Stop it!' as angrily as you can." She started out with a scream at the very top of her voice, which was shot through with fear. I coached her through the breathing she needed to keep going and to get her voice into a lower register, where the anger would vibrate through her. Once she connected with it strongly a few times, I had her lie down. I put my hands on her head and took her step by step through the surgery.

"It's a great privilege to be able to construct a woman's breast," Rebecca's plastic surgeon told me as he began the surgery. I was very impressed with his concern for her and the gentleness in the way he touched her. It was clear that she had told him at least some of her personal history and that it mattered to him. Before she went under, I got a feeling of a frightened child of about five or six and a pain and weeping in the area of her reconstructed left breast. The terror increased as the mask came down over her face. Once she was under, there was a feeling of nausea—another sign of fear.

When the surgeon started to work on the breast, I could feel rage in the chest wall. The transposed muscle seemed lonely and disoriented. No one had thanked it for leaving its comfortable place in Rebecca's back or encouraged and supported it in its new job of being part of her breast. I did it, making a note to tell Rebecca after the surgery how to talk to her muscle.

As the surgeon made the incision to remove the old implant and put in another, I got an image of something tumbling, over and over. It was a bundle of cells tumbling down a fallopian tube. I realized that Rebecca was reexperiencing the journey from the place of her conception in her mother's fallopian tube to the place of her implantation in the wall of her mother's uterus. It struck me that women who opt for breast implants are possibly trying to reactivate feelings about their own embryological implantation. My thoughts were interrupted by the surgeon saying, "Just watch this, Julie. It's like seeing your own adolescence in stop-time photography."

I watched Rebecca's breast swell in front of me, as the surgeon pumped saline solution into the new implant. I felt her pain and confusion at the time of her adolescence—sensations of desire, humiliation, and pride in her attractiveness and sexuality all mixed together. Was reactivating this adolescent turmoil another part of what implant surgery was about? At that moment I got an image of Rebecca looking about thirteen or fourteen, turning away from someone who was reaching for her breast. I felt her trying to go more unconscious under the anesthesia and got another image of a baby twisting and pulling away from someone. "Your body is for your own pleasure," I told her.

Looking at the unnaturally smooth surface of Rebecca's new breast, I asked the plastic surgeon when he would be reconstructing the nipple—and got a very strong message from Rebecca's body that the meaning of the missing nipple was "I can't nurture," which was passed down to her from her mother.

As he started to work on her back, the memory of being beaten came up very strongly. I got a feeling of the body trying to push the pain out with the scar tissue, to pretend that it had never penetrated Rebecca's being, that she had never really been hurt by it. When it was scraped and redressed, there was a feeling of relief and exhaustion. At the end of the surgery the anesthesiologist made a point of telling me that he had been able to go very light on the anesthesia, probably because of the work I was doing.

In the recovery room Rebecca was sobbing. She was also nauseated, as I thought she might be from the way she went under. Her nausea was probably a response to the terror reactivated by the surgery. "It really was very scary," I told her. "You were right to be scared. But it's over now, and you're safe," I said over and over again. I kissed her forehead and held her hand, allowing the waves of her terror to move through me. How nurtured I was by being able to offer someone a caring and watchful presence!

When I met with her for a postoperative session, I told her about my image of her breast being fondled by some man during her early adolescence, and she told me that an uncle had groped her. We did more anger release work, this time directed at her mother, who had been a controlling and vindictive force in her life and had done nothing to protect her from her uncle's abuse.

Permission Not to Have It

Like Grace, Rebecca had thought of herself as having both a healthy and a spiritual lifestyle, and she did not understand how she could possibly have become a victim of this disease. Our work together began to answer that question, I believe, by opening areas of pain and rage that needed to be addressed and giving her some tools for doing it. You cannot bypass your emotions on the way to health or spirituality and fully arrive there.

My next patient, Lorna, had been determined to avoid a mastectomy at all costs and had found the one surgeon in the San Francisco area willing to take off only a quarter of what she had been told was a seriously diseased breast, rather than the whole thing. In our preoperative session she told me about her abusive and alcoholic husband, her emotionally disturbed and demanding children, and her surgical history, which included twelve abortions. There was, predictably, sorrow in the area of her uterus, and rage at her mother at the site of a lumpectomy scar. She told me emphatically, however, that she was not angry at anyone.

The pathology report from the quadrectomy revealed that a mastectomy would be necessary. Lorna told me that she would rather commit suicide than lose her breast. "Would you feel the same way if it were a foot?" I asked.

"No," she told me. "But I used to be an artist's model. My breasts were famous. They are an essential part of who I am." She was in tears.

"Since you would commit suicide if you lost one, then you might as well not have the surgery and die of breast cancer," I told her. She appeared shocked. I was apparently the first person who had supported her in not having the surgery.

"Isn't there any alternative?" she asked.

"You might start by getting out of your marriage to an alcoholic husband, cleaning up your diet, and get to your anger," I told her. "But you've given me at least fifteen reasons why you can't do any of those things. So just don't have the surgery, and let nature take its course."

"But the people in my support group keep telling me I have to have it."

"If you don't like what they're telling you, find another support group." She was clearly not prepared for this. She looked at me, took a deep breath, and wiped tears off her cheeks.

"Do you know anything about tram flap reconstructions? Because that's what I'd like to have," she said, apparently able to entertain the idea of the surgery now that someone had given her permission not to have it. Remembering Andrea's surgery (in Chapter 9), a shudder ran through me. "How many abortions did you say you've had?"

"Twelve," she said. "I've had twelve abortions."

"Some women who opt for trams do so, I think, because unconsciously they want to reactivate the feelings in their wombs and their ovaries about those experiences. I think you might want to do the work now of letting go of the spirits of those children and then see how you feel about that particular surgery." She agreed but never called me again.

RESPONSIBILITY AND BLAME

One of the people I became friendly with in San Francisco (Belinda, the woman who had sent Lorna to me) was a social worker who was now involved in research about alternative therapies and breast cancer. Just about every time we met, she argued with me about the role of suppressed emotion in the disease. "How can you be so sure it plays a role?" she asked. My very certainty was clearly part of what irked her.

"All my work is intuitive, and this is what my gut tells me," I responded. "Look, if I ever meet a perfectly happy woman who had a wonderful, loving, nurturing childhood and also has breast cancer, I'll have to change my mind. But either they don't exist, or I just don't get to meet them." I knew this statement was extreme, but all my experience was leading me there. Hidden childhood sorrow just kept spilling out of my patients. "In any case, no one has ever been willing to put up any money to test my thesis and to see what a year of really deep emotional work, including prenatal and neonatal trauma work, might accomplish. No one's ever done it with a group of breast cancer patients and then, five years down the road, compared them with matched controls for survival rates. It's never been given a shot, so no one knows if I'm right or not."

While holding to her idea that my theory was "too simple" and that it's "much more complicated than that," she agreed. "But I still hate this idea of blaming people for their disease."

"First of all, you can hardly be blamed for something you didn't know anything about. That's what I tell my patients. How can you blame yourself for weakening your body by suppressing emotions, when you had no idea what effect it was having on you? And where were you supposed to find the support to be in touch with your feelings, when our society, in the name of 'productivity' or 'maturity,' emphasizes the very opposite? You'd have to go against a cultural norm. Achieving emotional intactness is a revolutionary act.

"Secondly, once you do realize what you've been doing to yourself, there's a difference between responsibility and blame. You can take responsibility for what you've done without hating yourself for it. In fact, you can have compassion for someone who felt forced to make such unhealthy choices. It's not about blame. On the contrary, it's about forgiveness and empowerment: forgiving yourself for what you've done, understanding why you did it, and feeling the power of being able to do something different."

As I continued to work with breast cancer patients, what interested me most was the potential for personal transformation that the disease represented in people's lives. In fact, I came to think of the so-called "crisis" in health care as an opportunity for the whole culture to heal on a level that had never occurred before.

The failure to "cure" chronic disease, along with chronic violence, is the great Achilles' heal of our ever-improving technological society. Disease, moreover, affects every level of society—every gender, every race, and every class. It is a universal summons to change. What I was working toward was to make healing a universal summons to honor and understand feeling.

Only when we acknowledge that our emotions—our fear, our anger, our pain, and our love—are our true guides to health, and our connection to each other and to the universe, will things change. For myself, the challenge was to understand in greater and greater depth how these forces operated in cells and even in molecules from the moment of conception, and perhaps even before.

HANDS OF PAIN

Some women opt for a "prophylactic" mastectomy—the removal of a nondiseased breast or breasts because the woman believes there is a serious threat that cancer will start there, often because of family history. It seemed to me utterly insane, a meaningless sacrifice that the medical profession had succeeded in terrorizing women into making. I now believe that no choice is meaningless for either the patient, the physician, or the society as a whole, but I was horrified when a young woman who had recently given birth came to me to prepare for such a surgery.

Lynn was also having a modified radical mastectomy on the other breast, which was diseased; had she not been, I might have refused to work with her altogether. The surgeon himself had advised against the prophylactic mastectomy, on the grounds that the disease was so virulent, she would have to be hit with the kind of chemotherapy that would either knock out the cancer completely or prove totally ineffective against its rampage through her body. The removal of the healthy breast was clearly her choice, and as we spoke, it seemed to fit into a sacrificial pattern playing out in her life.

Lynn, with her smooth unlined face, deep-set brown eyes, and hairless head from radiation treatments, looked very much like a baby herself when she sat down to talk with me. My first gentle suggestion that an absence of nurturing in her own life might be part of what had made her breast tissue so vulnerable to disease was greeted with a quick denial. "I had a very happy childhood. My parents were strict but very loving," she said. She did admit, however, that she lived in her husband's shadow, accommodating his wishes at every turn ahead of her own, and that the excessive time he spent away from home because of his work left her lonely and troubled. She also said that when she tried to discuss this with him, he didn't seem to understand what was bothering her. These admissions came after her assertion that they had a wonderful marriage.

I sensed a tremendous anger inside Lynn, but she seemed to have no avenue through which it could be released. "I believe in God and in forgiveness," she said when she lay down to start the energy work, "and I want more than anything else to live so I can take care of my daughter." She began to cry, but rage, not sorrow, emanated from her as she said this.

"Lynn, would you like to see your daughter treated by a

man the way your husband treats you, when she grows up and gets married?" I asked.

"No!" she said emphatically, clearly horrified.

"Then you might want to at least consider modeling a different kind of behavior for her, because that's how children learn—by example. You might consider standing up for yourself so she will know how to do it. You might consider getting angry about the things that have happened to you."

Lynn agreed, without getting up, to try to voice some of her anger. "Just say 'I'm angry!'" I told her, positioning myself at her feet to ground the energy. Her assertions of anger were very soft, almost whispered, at first, and floods of tears came from her eyes. I instructed her to think of her baby daughter and what she would do to anyone who tried to hurt her, and to say it more forcefully. This worked energetically, and she gave a few forceful blasts, before seeming to collapse in terror back into herself at the sound and force of her own voice.

"That was great," I said. "The purpose of blame, by the way, is not to stay focused on the person who hurt you, but to use it as an engine to mobilize your anger, and move forward with it. Then you can forgive. But blame serves a very real and necessary function as a step along the way, and you can't skip over it. There's nothing 'unspiritual' about blame as part of a process, or anger as an emotion that carries you forward into action. The end is always understanding and then love, but you can't just will yourself there. One of the reasons for having a body is to experience the path of this process. Otherwise, whoever or whatever created us could have just left us in the form of pure spirit or soul and let it go at that. The process is an elaboration, an expansion of love—an extension of spirit."

I was drawn to put my hand on Lynn's chest, just over the thymus gland, which plays a central function in the immune system. "I see you as a very little girl and quite forlorn," I said, "quite without defenses."

"I could never understand why my mother wouldn't stop drinking, even when I begged her," Lynn said. Just half an hour before, she had insisted she had a "happy childhood." I wondered what other hidden sorrows she was carrying in her wasted body.

On the day of the surgery, I met Lynn's parents, who had traveled out from the Northeast to be with her. Their concern and their love for her showed clearly in their faces, and I wondered what tortures of their own had kept them from connecting with Lynn in a more nurturing way when she was a child. Where in this chain of disconnection, abuse, and humiliation, passed down from parent to child, could a healer like myself most effectively intervene? I had the sense that most of my work with surgical patients was too little and came too late—not for their satisfaction but for my own.

A photographer from a national publication was in the operating room; he told me later how hard it was for him to see someone so young having this kind of surgery. "I thought about all my women friends and how vulnerable they are to this disease," he said. "I almost had to leave."

I felt fear rising in Lynn as soon as she went under, quickly crystallizing as the terror of a small child. As the surgeon cut deeper into the right breast, the one with the cancer, rage came up, which seemed to be associated with Lynn's adolescence. When the breast was removed, there was tremendous sorrow—a profound feeling of missing someone or something very precious, like the mother who was too busy drinking to be involved with her daughter. When the right breast was off the body, the surgeon started to work on removing the lymph nodes from under the adjacent arm for biopsying—and while he was working, he spoke with a colleague about scheduling difficulties and problems with an office manager. I had heard about surgeons discussing everything from stock market prices to golf scores while they were operating, but this was the first time I'd ever experienced it. I was shocked, and I could feel

Lynn's fury at being ignored. I leaned over to tell her that she was completely justified in her anger and that they should indeed be focusing on her and nothing else. I felt the tragic certainty that this inattention was recapitulating her experience as a child. When I felt the lymph nodes—most of which later turned out to be positive—there was the usual compacted rage I had come to expect in cancerous tissue.

The surgeon then started to remove the healthy left breast, and I felt a new level of rage in Lynn that seemed to connect with her preadolescence. There was also a feeling of sorrow and needless loss. Perhaps to distract myself from the horror of this mastectomy, I put myself inside the surgeon's hands to see what he was experiencing there. As if I were bringing my conscious awareness to some part of my own body, I said, "Be his hands, Julie." The first thing I felt was extreme pain, even agony, in the breast tissue he was handling. And then I felt waves of hostility shooting down his hands, starting at the wrist, with the very clear intention of blocking out the pain.

Again I was shocked. But before I knew what to do with this information, I started to feel very faint. I tried to steady myself, to ground my energy, but I could feel that at any moment I would be overwhelmed by the kind of sickening weakness that had come over me the very first time I watched open heart surgery. I left the operating room and stepped out into the sterile corridor. A nurse, reacting to the grayness of my complexion, got me a chair and suggested that I sit down, bend over, and let my head hang between my knees.

I did so, begging for it to be over and wondering, in my vanity, what the photographer must be thinking. Why was this happening to me now, I wondered, after more than thirty operations? The nurse put a wet, cool towel on my neck. After a few minutes I picked my head up. I tried to stand, but I was a little wobbly and sat down again in despair, wondering if Lynn felt I had abandoned her. A few minutes later, against the advice of the nurse, I got up and went back in. The surgeon was suturing the wound on the left side of Lynn's breast, and the moment I saw it, I felt faint again and had to leave.

A few minutes later, I went back in again as a nurse was finishing dressing the wound, and I felt fine. I apologized to Lynn, who was still unconscious, stayed with her to the end of the surgery, then accompanied her to the recovery room.

Had it been the horror of seeing a healthy breast removed that triggered such a strong reaction? But if so, why would I have had it again, just as strongly, when the surgeon's hands were closing the wound—and not when the nurse was dressing it? Susan Osborne had said healers seem to "take in" bad feelings when a healing situation triggers an issue that you haven't dealt with yet. It must have been the hostility in the surgeon's hands blocking out Lynn's pain, I concluded, that set me off.

Abusive parents actually enjoy hitting their children—it gives them physical release from the anger or fear they can't tolerate or contain. Just as Lynn's surgeon was unaware of his own hostility toward her helplessness and her pain, parents are unaware of the hostility or terror that their children's vulnerability evokes in them. Once they discharge the feeling into the child's body, they no longer experience it. In fact, they often can't remember it, and when the child sulks afterward, they seem perplexed, as if nothing has happened. This was certainly my experience when hit as a child, and clearly I had unresolved feelings about my helplessness in those situations. I thought, too, of the invasions of my body by my sexual abusers. Clearly I had more healing work to do on myself in this area.

People become surgeons for many different reasons, and the same specialty—even the same surgery—can be used to satisfy a wide range of emotional needs. Would I ever dare bring this up for discussion with surgeons themselves? I wondered. Probably not, if I wanted to continue to work with them.

My next surgery was a mastectomy with a tram flap reconstruction. The patient, Loretta, told me she had suffered sexual abuse and grown up in an alcoholic family. Memories of the abuse and a feeling of rage during intercourse came up when the plastic surgeon made the incision for the tram over Loretta's uterus and ovaries. Unlike the tram flap surgery in New York, in which the plastic surgeon waited for the mastectomy to be completed before beginning his work, here the two occurred almost simultaneously, making for much shorter time under anesthesia. I decided to slip into the general surgeon's hands and found, to my relief, that they were full of compassion, meeting the pain coming from the patient's body with wave after wave of tenderness. I then entered the plastic surgeon's hands and felt a rush of nausea. His hands were up by the patient's breast at the time; when they were down at her pelvis, there were feelings of great tenderness. Did this difference reflect the surgeon's feelings, respectively, about nurturing and sexuality, and how his own parents might have related to him around these issues? I didn't feel comfortable discussing it. Nor did I mention how uncomfortable the patient seemed with the loud music that accompanied the completion of the surgery.

To Speak or Not to Speak

Usually I was so sensitive to the fact that I was serving at the sufferance of the surgeons that I didn't voice any objections to what I observed in the operating room. Nor did I usually mention it to the patients afterward, unless they pressed me by asking very specific questions. If they seemed happy with the experience, I didn't feel it was my place to volunteer information that would send them back into the surgeon's office with troubling questions.

I admit that this was cowardly. It would probably have been better to ask a patient up front, "If I see or sense anything I don't like happening during the surgery, do you want me to tell you about it afterward?" But in the rush of getting through the twenty cases I had committed to doing, it didn't occur to me.

In one situation, however, I was so appalled by what was said in the OR that I had to speak up, and in another I actually did share with the patient how I felt about what had happened.

Charlotte was a large, gentle-looking woman with a great deal of sorrow in her eyes, which stayed there even when she smiled. She was scheduled for a mastectomy with a saline implant reconstruction on one side and a breast reduction on the other. Although she was troubled and frightened by the disease, her breasts were large to the point of physical discomfort, and she was also looking forward to having the smaller breasts she had always wanted. In our pre-op session she told me that about a year before her diagnosis of breast cancer, her business had failed and that the humiliation was almost unbearable for her. She was still trying to pay back her creditors. Earlier on in her life, she had had an abortion under circumstances that were very upsetting to her and about which her feelings were still unresolved. "Some feelings about that might come up during the surgery," I said. "If they do, I'll be there to help you experience them in complete safety and release them."

When we finished with the preparation for the surgery, she told me that she had already been excited about the surgery because of the breast reduction, but now she felt the possibility that a truly profound healing could occur in the operating room as well. This was, of course, what I wished for her, so I was extremely upset by the banter that went on between the attending general surgeon and the young male resident who was working with him on the mastectomy part of the surgery.

Why is it so hard for some surgeons to remember what a significant event this operation is in a woman's life? What feelings are they avoiding by turning it into something so automatic and routine that discussions that have nothing to do with the person lying on the table can fly back and forth across her body? What cost involvement?

I felt Charlotte's rage at being ignored, and memories came

up in her of being five or six and having the same feeling. Then she settled into despair, with a particularly heavy feeling in the center of her chest. This is where the thymus gland, which plays a key role in the immune system, is located, so I associated the heaviness with a resigned feeling about not being able to defend herself. I did what I could to comfort her, then heard the resident asking the attending surgeon if he was going to remove the breast or take the lymph nodes out first. "I know you usually take the breast first, but you know, we could take the nodes first if we could get a hoist in here," he said, making a cruel and tasteless joke about the size of Charlotte's breast. I felt her rage at that, then her utter humiliation. There was also great sorrow as the breast left her body, which seemed to be her mother's sorrow. I told her that she would not have to carry that feeling for her mother any longer.

When the mastectomy was almost completed, the resident stripped off his gloves and said, "Whew! I'm glad that's over. Mastectomies give me the willies." It was everything I could do to keep from going for his throat. To my utter surprise, no one said a word.

As soon as he was out the door, I said to the attending surgeon, "Someone should talk to that young man about what he says during these surgeries."

"That's probably just his way of dealing with his discomfort," he said.

But I couldn't let it go. "That level of discomfort should be dealt with before he steps into an operating room, and if he can't resolve it, he shouldn't be working on mastectomies." I would like to think that I was simply voicing what everyone else in the room was thinking, but much more likely, if I hadn't said anything, his behavior would have gone unnoticed as well as uncommented upon.

When the implant was put in, there was a feeling in Charlotte's body of much misery and suffering as a fetus—a feeling of being unwanted and of implantation in her mother's womb being very difficult for her. Was the abortion she later had in part a reaction to these feelings?

As in a previous surgery we had done together, the plastic surgeon told me that the blood loss was surprisingly little, and Charlotte later reported that she regained the use of the arm from which the lymph nodes were taken much more quickly than expected. This news interested me much less than the psychological drama of the surgical experience, although details of effectiveness on a physical level are more likely to make energy healing a popular practice during surgery.

Right after this one I had a case during which the surgeon was discussing other things almost from the moment she "cut skin." In our post-op session the patient mentioned to me how put off she was by the surgeon's coldness and apparent lack of personal concern for her when she visited her in her office. "I had the same experience of her during surgery," I said. "It seemed to me that she was repeating the kind of treatment you got from your mother. She did what she had to do on a mechanical, physical level, but she didn't connect to you as a person."

"I suppose she has to be that way," the patient said, like a child rationalizing an unfeeling parent's behavior.

"Not at all. It's a choice. You deserve better."

The Myth of Detachment

According to a widespread myth, emotional involvement interferes with technical performance. But this myth completely ignores the way intellect, action, and feeling are related. In any field peak performance is about embracing a task with all of your energies, including your emotional energies. Exhaustion comes from struggling to deny what we are feeling.

According to a related myth, doctors do not become "emotionally involved with" or "attached to" their patients, because if they did, the pain of the illness and death they must deal with would overwhelm them. That is, they have to cut off their feelings in order to survive.

But many people turn to alternative healers in times of serious illness exactly because they are missing caring and personal commitment from the medical profession. Alternative healers who deal with cancer on a regular basis do not have to cut off their feelings.

Unfortunately, the bias against feeling in the operating room reflects the bias against feeling in our whole society. Being "emotional" is considered being "inefficient" or "nonobjective." The idea that the energy of emotion sharpens both physical and mental performance is quite alien to us. We still consider feelings in large part the province of women and therefore, like every aspect of this still second-class gender, irrelevant, weak, or inferior. In the light of this reality, how could I ever demonstrate to surgeons that being completely aware of what both they and their patients are feeling would actually enhance both performance and outcomes? The task seems overwhelming, but there are some small rays of hope.

Over the past several years I have spoken to students at medical schools, and each year I find greater interest in maintaining emotional intactness for themselves as physicians and in engaging in the emotional life of their patients. A student at Dartmouth, to my delight, asked me, "How could we use the kind of healing work you do preventatively with our patients?"

"If you, as their doctors, validate the importance of their feelings in maintaining their health," I replied, "it will have a tremendous effect."

Another ray of hope is an experiment currently being conducted in the United Kingdom by a pediatric cardiac surgeon. He had performed a number of very difficult surgeries with no mortality, then had seven deaths in his next ten cases. Appalled, he went over the circumstances of each case and decided that the critical factor might have been the emotional relationships among the staff during the surgery. He is now formally studying the connection between how people working in the operating room relate to each other and surgical outcomes.

Finally, patients themselves may begin evaluating surgeons and other physicians in terms of the depth of their emotional connection with them, and sharing those evaluations. Most miraculously, doctors, along with other authority figures, may be tiring of the role into which we have thrust them. Just as it is becoming more and more acceptable for fathers to openly adore and be involved with their children, so it may become more acceptable for doctors to show the flood of feeling that they must experience at the trust and vulnerability of their patients.

A key part of this shift will be medical training itself. The devastating role it plays in wiping out the life of feeling became starkly apparent to me during a day-long retreat for interns and residents at a hospital in the Bay Area. First of all, the thirty-odd young men and women who came were the most exhausted and unhealthy-looking bunch of people in their twenties I had ever seen. How are such people supposed to support the life-force in their patients? I wondered. We did an exercise in which each of us had to choose two words, one to describe how we were and another to describe how we would like to be. I was horrified at what they said about themselves: insecure, depressed, unhappy, incompetent. Why were they uniformly feeling so bad about themselves? Why wasn't anybody more concerned about it?

I am certainly not the first person to observe that the grinding down of character, individuality, and self-worth that often occurs in medical training is counterproductive and unnecessary. Considering how overworked people who study medicine are and how little attention is given to their own emotional and even physical needs, it is something of a miracle that they emerge with even a shred of compassion and energy left over for their patients, as indeed some of them do.

But their training constantly reminds them that they are there to perform a series of technical tasks and nothing more. In part this message has to do with the idea that their job is to "do battle" with a disease rather than to engage in a healing relationship with the patient. Internship and residency in particular smack of military training.

Parenting has gradually been changing in our country because of the commitment of people to go back and experience their own pain growing up, to avoid passing it on to their children; we will also need a generation of physicians who have not been brainwashed into thinking that sleep deprivation and emotional suppression have made them better doctors. Only people willing to admit how badly and needlessly they have been hurt by the system can muster the anger and the clarity to change it, rather than perpetuate it.

Chapter Thirteen

⌁

THE VIOLENCE
OF MEDICINE

As I continued to do breast cancer surgeries, I encountered over and over again the buried rage of women who have suffered neglect, abandonment, hostility, and physical and sexual abuse. Of the female private patients I saw, the disease or discomfort in every one of them was connected to a humiliation inflicted upon them as girls and repeated in some form as adults. I could spend virtually all my time as a healer, I realized, just helping people express that initial out-of-control rage from childhood that blocks the flow of so much other feeling and action in their lives.

I talked to Sonja Gilligan about this problem, and we toyed with the idea of setting up "anger clinics," where releasing anger would be the focus. Of course other feelings are also blocked. But when you consider that control of anger is how parents control their children—in fact, how all people in positions of authority control those beneath them in the hierarchy—you begin to understand just how powerful a device allowing people to experience and own their anger can be.

One problem in getting people to understand this connection is the confusion about the relationship between anger and violence. People who are in touch with their anger, who are clear about how they have been hurt and by whom, do not have to be violent. The very experience of the anger moving through their bodies gives them the sensation of being powerful and intact. It also clears their mind and gives them information about how to act—how to name what has happened to them with clarity, and how to move on.

People who are violent (like the many mass murderers who the neighbors say were such "nice guys") are people who do not feel their anger and have buried their pain. In fact, violent acts themselves are a way of getting anger out of the body, without ever owning it. Violent people are people who have been hurt and humiliated, often violently, with no recourse of protecting themselves or protesting. Intact anger would bring up a memory of the wound, which is part of what they are avoiding.

When they are poor, without social or economic power, they often explode in violent acts, not against their primary aggressors, their parents, but against someone who shows them a much milder form of disrespect, in reality or in imagination. When they are middle class, they often turn the violence against their own bodies.

The taboo against a child's owning her anger and the control exerted by this taboo is so pervasive that we hardly even notice it. Commands like "Don't look at me like that!" or "Don't talk like that to your mother!" are rarely thought of as child abuse—any more than hitting a child was twenty years ago. To understand the force of the degradation being imposed in these situations, however, we need only imagine how we would feel if these commands were addressed to us as adults, by someone twice or three times our size, with complete physical power over us.

(I am always tempted, when I visit parents at mealtime who are telling their kids that they must "eat everything on their plates," to ask how they would feel if their hostess made the same demand when they were at a dinner party.)

It is not surprising, therefore, that even under anesthesia patients often try to suppress their anger, going more unconscious when great rage comes up in them. After all, they are in the hands of someone who has the power of life and death over them, as their parents once did.

The last surgery I worked in before leaving San Francisco was another mastectomy with a tram flap reconstruction, and once again the patient had had an abortion. Georgette, a lovely, gentle, soft-spoken woman in her late forties, had also given a child up for adoption, and part of the work we did before the surgery was having her let go of the energies of those two children, which I felt were still attached to her and needed to be released.

"Tell them how sorry you are that you couldn't keep them, and let them go with love," I said. "They will understand. They've been waiting to hear this from you, and when you release them, they will be free to incarnate at a better time and in a better place. This is your gift to them."

The insertion of the breathing tube brought up terror in Georgette, accompanied by memories of abuse that were heightened when the Foley catheter was put in her urethra and that seemed to go back to the ages of three and four. The often insensitive insertion of tubes and catheters into the supposedly insensate bodies of abuse victims must bring up a whole world of trauma, I thought. I put my hand on her lower abdomen to calm her and felt all the fear from her first two pregnancies rippling through her. The swabbing of her body with betadine brought up the memory of being bathed as a baby, and the first incision sent her into a state of despairing submission.

When the lymph nodes were removed from her arm, I got the feeling of a little child's being yanked along by an adult, as I had so often before. The cutting of the nipple brought up all her mother's pain and bitterness at nursing her, and I told her to release them from her body.

The plastic surgeon became concerned when the venous blood flow in the flap that she was bringing up from the lower abdomen to form a breast had stopped. This stoppage, which could cause the tissue to die, was often a problem in these surgeries. The information that came to me from Georgette's body was that she didn't want the memory of the abortion that was in this tissue to reach her heart. She didn't want to connect to her anger about it because she was afraid, growing up in a violent family, that she herself would do something violent. "Georgette," I leaned over and said, "I want you to love the young woman who had to make that decision. And I want this feeling of loving yourself for having the abortion to come into the right atrium of your heart." As I said this, the flap began to regain its normal healthy color.

When the second breast came off her body, a wave of nausea swept through Georgette, which carried both her mother's feeling of rejecting her as a child and her own feelings about giving up a child. Looking at the bloody mass of flesh with its wrinkled skin, I wondered as I often had before, at exactly what moment it stopped being a breast and became an object no longer attached in any way to a human body.

At the end of the surgery to reconstruct the second breast, I felt Georgette going more unconscious. Grounding myself by allowing my feet to draw energy up from the earth, I told her to come back. As with Barbara a year earlier in open heart surgery, she came back with what felt like a roar, and this time the rage brought with it memories of her own birth and the desire to fight through the anesthetized state of her mother's numbness and thrust herself out into the world. I told her that this surgery was indeed an opportunity for rebirth, with a new body and a new sense of herself within that body.

When we spoke a week after the surgery, Georgette told me that she had left the hospital earlier than expected and was not taking any pain medication. She also told me that she was feeling unafraid and very happy with herself.

One again I had been impressed by the depth and complexity of the surgical journey, and I wondered what was going on simultaneously in the energy memories of the surgeon. A French obstetrician once theorized that the reason people participating in medical births are so eager to anesthetize women is that they themselves are frightened by feelings about their own birth that are evoked. When I was working at Columbia, I had once told the head of the cardiothoracic surgery department that I thought it would be a good idea to put surgeons into trance and have them experience step by step each kind of surgery they have to perform as if they were the patient. "I think they would discover things about the surgery that would change and refine the way they work," I told him. Although he was open to the idea, we never got around to it.

I wanted to allow the surgeons to experience just what their patients were feeling and how a body reacts to each part of the surgical process. With their intimate knowledge of anatomy and physiology, I was convinced that the surgeons would discover subtleties at the tissue and even the cellular level that would help their technique. Now it occurred to me that it might reveal to them just what touching each part of the body stimulates in their own psyches, and that this would be useful and healing as well.

Healing Through Violence

While I was being given a tour of the chemotherapy treatment rooms at one of the Bay Area hospitals, looking at the patients with tubes of bright red liquid filled with toxic chemicals dripping into them, the full significance of chemotherapy and all its side effects hit me like a bolt of lightning. "Umbilical affect," I said to myself.

This term is used by prenatal psychologists to describe the response of a fetus to stress hormones and other toxic chemicals that come from the mother through the umbilical cord and enter the bloodstream as if the fetus itself had produced, inhaled, or ingested them. The memory of this affect in an adult often triggers an uncontrolled jerking of the pelvis. This hip jerking used to occur in me spontaneously whenever anyone doing bodywork on me touched me for the first time.

The movement is an unconscious attempt to thrust these chemicals away—to push them back into the mother. Photographs have been taken that show babies in utero grasping their umbilical cords so tightly with their hands, in order to stop the flow of toxicity into their bodies, that nothing can get through. After a while the lack of oxygen causes the heart rate to drop and the grip relaxes, but the fetus may do this repeatedly.

In another prenatal workshop I took, my partner palpated the area over my navel, holding her hand a couple of feet above my body, and my hips began to jerk violently. As she brought her hand closer to the surface of my body, I felt very frightened and violently ill. When I tried to push her hand away, at first it felt almost impossible. My arms felt weak and helpless. Then, as I kept breathing, I had an impulse to growl. Energy came flooding forward from a place in my upper back, an angry strength flooded into my arms, and I was able to push the hand up away from my body with ease.

Unquestionably I was reexperiencing and repatterning

Hands
of
Life

what had happened to me inside my mother's womb. All of a sudden my years of bulimia made sense. Here, embedded in my earliest experience of being nurtured, was the sensation that the nourishment itself was toxic. No wonder I'd had a love-hate relationship with food, wanting frantically to draw it into my body and just as frantically to expel it again. Umbilical affect might also explain my passivity during the childhood sexual abuse I suffered, about which I told no one: I had already had the experience of having something come into my body that I couldn't control and that was harmful to me. The shock from that trauma was probably retriggered by my sexual abusers.

Now, looking at the patients on chemo drips, it struck me that chemotherapy itself might recapitulate the experience of receiving chemical toxicity in the womb. After all, to the extent that it works, it does so because it is most lethal to cells that are dividing very quickly, at the rate of fetal cells. Moreover, these cells often have the primitive, undifferentiated quality of embryological or fetal cells.

If growth and protection are antagonistic functions in the body (and we know they are—you cannot defend yourself and grow at the same time, on either the cellular or the body level; your energy can be focused only on one of these functions at a time), then stress hormones coming into the fetal body could arrest cellular growth. Suppose this was exactly what happened in cancer patients' prenatal lives. When something in their adult lives evokes a strong enough memory of prenatal life, cells convert to that state of intense, urgent growth, and the patient seeks unconsciously to repeat the whole cycle by poisoning those cells to arrest their growth.

Where, then, would radiation come in? Because of its energetic quality, I began to think that radiation might recapitulate hostile thinking on the part of the mother or the father, which would be communicated, by de Broglie waves or by a low-level electromagnetic frequency, to the surface proteins of the fetus's cells, or directly to the electrochemical bonds in the DNA inside the cells' nuclei.

I discussed this idea with a breast cancer survivor who'd had surgery, chemotherapy, and radiation. "I can't tell you exactly why," she said, "but on a gut level it makes a lot of sense. I used to tell people when I was trying to describe my experience of chemo to them, 'It's like nothing else you've ever experienced, but it's strangely familiar.' What you've suggested, Julie, would explain that."

The idea that chemotherapy recapitulates umbilical affect and that radiation recapitulates hostile thinking during the pregnancy also made sense to me in terms of the medical profession's attachment to these often ineffective and damaging forms of treatment. Why, with all the millions spent in the "war on cancer" over all these years, was there such an intense, almost exclusive focus on these two forms of treatment? Why was the push almost always toward "better" chemotherapy agents and "more effective" kinds of radiation? Why weren't more people looking diligently in other directions? To me, the answer lay exactly in the symbolic meaning of these two treatments. They signify something that on an unconscious level both the medical profession and the public know about this disease: the violence of the treatment reevokes the violence of the initial condition that set the scene for triggering it.

Going Public

Shortly after this my sponsors at the Institute for Health and Healing asked me to address a gathering of present and potential funders on the general subject of energy medicine. Since it is my habit always to talk about what most excites me, I mentioned these ideas about prenatal factors in breast cancer in my talk, along with an explanation in terms of both physics and cellular biology, of some possible mechanisms through which energy healing works.

I described the more general idea that the nervous system works in many ways we don't understand and that energy healing may simply be utilizing one or more of those yet-to-be-explained pathways of communication between and within cells. I talked about this and my surgical protocols at surgical grand rounds early one morning at California Pacific, the medical center in which the institute is housed. I discussed my ideas about prenatal influences on disease and my discovery that patients relive old trauma during surgery—including trauma from life in the womb.

Shortly after my talk, I got a call from Bill Stewart, an ophthalmologist at California Pacific, the medical director of the institute and one of its original founders. "Julie," he told me, "I thought the talk you gave was excellent, and I particularly appreciated your scientific explanation of what you do. But you said some things that were really upsetting and that I know doctors were uncomfortable with. It's all that prenatal stuff. Couldn't you just leave it out? It really spoils the very wonderful sense you present of yourself as a serious and scientific person."

Where had I heard this before? My mind flashed back to the early days of working with Dr. Oz: *"You know, your work with the patients is really wonderful, and they respond to you so well. But do you have to use the word energy? It's so far outside the scientific model or anything that anyone here could understand. Can't you just say you're rubbing their feet?"* Sure, I thought to myself—and can't you just say you're rubbing their chests when they come in for open heart surgery?

Now, of course, three years later, everybody was talking about energy, and energy healers were out of the closet. I wondered if three years from now everybody would be talking about prenatal factors in chronic disease and regressive states under anesthesia. I didn't, however, voice this thought to Dr. Stewart, whom I liked tremendously and who had labored to make the institute viable when few other doctors at the medical center had taken any interest in it. I knew that he was expressing a genuine concern that my attachment to "far out" ideas would jeopardize my credibility with the medical staff, and that his impulse toward me was protective.

"This is hard for me, Bill," I told him, "because it's what I believe. I can't not talk about it. Even when I leave it out of my lectures, it inevitably comes up through a question someone asks about the work. But if you could think of a way to make these ideas more palatable to your colleagues or direct me to some other kind of language to use, I'd be very grateful." This was really my responsibility, not his, and I resolved, in my nonexistent free time, to study embryology and see if I could make more medically persuasive arguments for my point of view.

When I undertook that study, I discovered that embryology was not a subject to which a great deal of attention was given in medical school. "You sort of inhale that course," an intern friend told me. This made me wonder if perhaps many unsolved medical mysteries had their roots in this period of greatest change, greatest learning, most rapid growth, and greatest vulnerability—when the body is first learning how to be a body, and the brain is learning the vast majority of what it will know about being a brain.

The California Pacific Cardiac Patients' Group

I introduced some of these ideas, along with some general principles of energy healing, to the group I was running at California Pacific for cardiac patients. Like the patients at Columbia, the group members were shy and engaging with, for the most part, little exposure to alternative ideas. I asked them to begin by drawing or writing a description of their hearts in a way that was expressive of how their hearts felt to them. For most of them it was the first time they had thought about having a conscious relationship with this organ beyond worrying how it might fail them. A number of them told me that they didn't think they could do the exercise at first, but then they were surprised by the words, images, and movements that came out of them—how much they knew and how deeply they felt about their hearts. I was particularly moved by the drawings of Maria, who had suffered a heart attack a year and three months after her daughter was stabbed in the heart and killed by an irate lover. One showed a large but incomplete heart, with no point at its bottom. On the top she wrote the words "Prayer" and "Love" and, over in one corner, "Scars to Stars." But at the bottom, very large, where the point should have been, there were "Tears," "Blood," and "Anger."

The essential emotional energy of the heart, I explained to the group, is not love but anger—the forward, aggressive, throbbing movement of blood through the body. In fact, I said, this is the characteristic energy of all healthy muscle tissue. "When you say 'Take heart,' you mean 'Have courage,' not 'Be more loving.' And the very word 'courage,' which suggests aggressive boldness, comes from the French word for the heart, *le coeur.*

"Love is the energy of the sac of connective tissue that surrounds and protects the heart, the pericardium. We usually think of anger as protecting love, but the softness of love can form a protective shield around the vulnerable action of anger as well." I then had them divide into pairs, with one person being the heart and the other the pericardium. I instructed the "hearts" to tell the "pericardia" exactly what they needed for comfort and protection, and the pericardia to give it to them. Then I had them reverse roles. It turned out to be a wonderful device to get them to share their needs, fears, and desires with each other and to strengthen the bonds of connection among them. It also allowed them to feel and understand the work of these organs on a nonintellectual level and to observe how their emotional attitudes about protecting themselves and receiving protection were affecting them physically.

The next week I introduced them to the idea that although the overriding energy of the heart is anger or forward, aggressive movement, each chamber within the heart carries the energy of a different emotion. This was something I discovered one day by going into each of the chambers of my own heart and sensing the emotional energy there.

"The left atrium, which takes in oxygen and with it information from the outside world via the lungs, carries the energy of fear, excitement, and perception. The left ventricle, which is the largest chamber, whose contractions you experience as your 'heart beat,' and which sends the oxygenated blood with its nourishment and information coursing through the body, carries the energy of anger, or forward movement. It also carries the protective energy of anger, since this blood carries the cells and the chemicals of the immune system to all parts of the body. The right atrium, which draws blood through the veins back into the heart, carries the energy of pain and self-knowledge. Venous blood, carrying gases and waste materials out of the cells, also carries information about the cells, and about the body itself, back to the heart. The right ventricle, which sends the venous blood back to the lungs, which release carbon dioxide back into the atmosphere to nourish plants and trees, carries the energy of love and connection out from ourselves to others."

I then led them in a meditation in which I had them imagine each chamber of the heart in turn. "See it, and now step inside it as if it were a room. Notice its color and its texture and ask yourself, 'How old am I here? What kind of person am I in this chamber of my heart?' " I had done this exercise once before at a workshop in Boulder. One of the participants had an insight into her asthma through realizing how cramped and dark her left atrium, which draws blood back from the lungs, felt to her. By working on consciously expanding that chamber, she found could relieve her symptoms.

When I asked my cardiac patients to share about their experience, they all expressed surprise at how different each chamber felt and the different ages they associated with them. "I think that those ages represent times when something happened with your experience of the emotion carried in that chamber," I told them. "I think that the memory of it is still there and needs to be released. If a chamber felt particularly cramped or uncomfortable for you, you might think of what you would have to do to expand it and make it more welcoming, both in your mind and in your life." As a device to help, I suggested that when they went home, they assign a different room in their house to represent each of the four chambers. I told them that I wanted them to put an object in each one that represented how they felt about that chamber and to spend at least a few minutes every day meditating on the chamber while standing in that room.

In another session I introduced them to the idea that how their parents felt about their conception, gestation, and birth might have had a major effect on their hearts. The heart is the first organ to be formed in utero, and it starts to beat in the third week after conception, just around the time when there is usually medical confirmation of the pregnancy. "How your parents felt about the pregnancy came into your awareness just as your heart started to beat," I said. I also discussed with them the fact that in the womb the circulatory pattern insures that the most highly oxygenated blood goes to the upper body and the brain. "If this has been a traumatic period for you," I say, "I think that energetically this pattern of focusing on the upper body and the brain remains after birth, even though the circulation changes."

I then had them lie down, and I led them meditatively through their conception, gestation, and birth, describing in detail what was happening with their hearts and their circulation at each step. Some of them fell asleep, some were moved to tears, and some got a very clear sense of what their parents were feeling and their reaction to those feelings each step of the way. "I didn't like that," one of them told me when it was over. "It was so depressing. I felt so lonely."

"That's one of the feelings your heart has been holding for you all these years," I said. "It's time to think about bringing it into full consciousness, experiencing it, and letting it go."

I have done this kind of regressive meditation, using various breathing techniques and suggestions to allow people to drift back to their origins, many times now, and I never cease to be amazed at the amount of information that comes through. Bruce Lipton believes that memory precedes the formation of the nervous system—that it is held in the cell membrane in the reactive responses of the surface proteins. My own experience with this exercise would certainly suggest that he is right.

One problem in working with such ideas with people who have very serious and advanced illness, like many of my cardiac and cancer patients, is that they have already gone to extreme measures to keep painful or disruptive memories out of their consciousness. They have somatized things to such a degree that reversing the habit can be extremely difficult, particularly when they are not convinced of the value of doing so. The real barrier, however, is not lack of intellectual conviction but terror. They honestly feel that they are fighting back the only way they can. They still dread the parental penalty for feeling their feelings, especially their anger, clearly. They become trapped in the revenge of self-destruction.

In this respect they are in sync with a society that refuses to see connections between the humiliation it inflicts upon its racial minorities and its poor, and the self-destructive epidemics of violence that spring from those populations and eventually threaten us all. Nor collectively do we understand that our abuse of the planet that nurtures us comes from our humiliated longing for nurturing.

Probably my most startling experience in the operating room came with Christina, a very pretty woman in her early forties who was scheduled for a lumpectomy with an axillary node dissection (removal of a lump from the breast for both curative and diagnostic purposes and removal of lymph nodes from the breast and under the arm). She wore beautiful, exotic clothes, flowing scarves, and unusual, custom-designed jewelry, and had the external confidence of the attractive woman that she was.

But her underlying shadow of self-doubt made me want to hug her and comfort her. She was yet another woman who told me that she had led an exemplarily healthy lifestyle and couldn't understand why this was happening to her body. She had renewed her devotion to her spiritual practice of prayer and meditation, she said, and was also working regularly with a bodyworker, an energy healer, and a hypnotherapist. She had just come back from swimming with dolphins off the Florida coast.

All this work had not served to assuage her sense of profound isolation. Her mother, she told me, had not been very interested in children and treated her own as something of an inconvenience. Christina had had the misfortune to be born after a stillbirth and another infant who had died when only a few days old. Her parents' marriage was an unhappy one, and when she was very young, her father left for the war. Her marriage too had been unhappy. She told me with great sorrow that she didn't know if she would ever be able to attract and sustain a connection with the kind of man with whom she would like to have an intimate relationship.

"You believe that in order to be who you are, you have to be alone," I said. "It's not true, of course. But you certainly couldn't be who you were around your mother. Her promise was that if you just subordinated yourself to her and looked after her needs, eventually you would get taken care of. The problem is that that taking care of never happened for you, and you're furious about it." I suggested to Christina that she do an anger exercise of putting her mother on the wall and blasting her with the word "Traitor." Very quickly a volcano of rage erupted from her, followed by a sweet, painful feeling of self-knowing.

The pain of valuing herself was so potent that I suggested she do another exercise, also borrowed from my encounter group days: "I want you to take a deep breath, and as you exhale, say, 'I know my daddy loved me.'" After she did this for a while, the pain was transformed into a warm, glowing feeling of love. I had her continue, dipping back into the pain and feeling the love again. "This was the feeling that your mother never wanted you to have and that will allow you to bring that man into your life and keep him there," I told her.

As she was talking about herself, the depth of her despair had been so profound that I felt a need to take her back to its roots—her prenatal life. But I first needed to know how far back in her existence her belief system would allow her to go. "Do you believe that we exist in some energetic form, before we exist as bodies?" She told me that she did. "Good, because that's where we're going to start. If you didn't, I wasn't going to ride roughshod over your belief system and insist on taking you there."

I myself was not completely sold on the idea of a spiritual existence preceding or following our material one. But a couple of experiences had inclined me in that direction, and I was now willing to give it a little more than the benefit of the doubt. The first of these experiences was at the end of some energy work I did with Kim Brady, my teacher at Kripalu. When we reached the end of the session, I found myself saying, still lying on his table, "I'm not going to die when I die." This was the kind of language I would normally be embarrassed about, but at the time it made perfect energetic sense. "I feel as if there is no time, and that I am everywhere at once," I said, and then, with a great sigh and a feeling of supreme exultation, "I am without expectation."

Indeed, I had no sense of either body or intellect at that point. I felt as if I were made entirely of light and coextensive with the entire universe. If we do survive at all, I realized (although after the effects of the session wore off, I began to doubt this), it is with neither flesh nor thought. We are simply pure energy, like light—all over space in a single moment, which is also every possible moment. There also isn't any "I" to it—just pure existence, with no hint of personality.

My other intimation of a spiritual existence apart from a physical one came in a meditation similar to the one I was about to do with Christina, which I experienced in one of William Emerson's workshops. He had asked us to be ourselves as we were before we were born. Immediately the sense of being a spinning vortex of energy came over me. Whether this represented who or what I actually was or just the will and energy of my parents on the way to creating me, I had no idea. But it felt powerful and real to me at the time.

I asked Christina to lie down and to begin by just noticing her breathing. Then I had her breathe as if air were coming in through her navel. "Now I want you to try a different kind of breathing," I said. "This is the breathing of the cells. It is the breath beneath the breath—the breathing that goes on, even when you hold your breath. Just as the lungs take in oxygen and give off carbon dioxide and other waste gases, so does every cell in your body. Just feel that now—the simple but insistent breathing of the cells." This was a technique I learned from Bonnie Cohen. As I spoke, I had my hands on Christina's feet and was attuning the movement of my diaphragm to the pace of my own cellular breathing. This created both the safety and the model for Christina to do the same. I usually do these meditations with my hands on the feet or the head, depending on whether the person needs more to be grounded or to feel a direct brain connection with what I'm saying.

"This is the breathing that began at the moment of your conception," I said, "but the rhythm is much older than that. It is a fundamental pulsing of the universe. So when you breathe, you breathe the universe." I didn't know exactly what I meant by this, but I had discovered long ago that much of healing is poetry and that I have to trust the words that come to me.

I felt Christina go into a state of deep relaxation, and then, sensing her to have an energy pattern very similar to my own, I gave her the image that had come to me during my own regression. "I want you to experience yourself as you were before you were born. I want to feel yourself as pure energy—as a spinning vortex of energy out in the universe with all the other energy spirits. Just see how it feels to you. How you like this state of being pure energy." She smiled.

"Now I want you to see and feel yourself in time and in space getting closer to the moment of your birth. See yourself getting closer and closer to the planet Earth. And see the planet as it was in the year that you were conceived. Also see your parents and anyone else who was present in your family at that time.

"Say good-bye now to all the other spirits, and listen very carefully to what they have to tell you—their parting words as you leave." Christina looked distressed, and I interrupted the meditation to ask her what was going on.

"I don't want to do it," she said. "I don't want to go there." This is a common response from people who have experienced a great deal of pain in their lives. Whether it is hindsight or an actual memory of the agony of spirit entering flesh, I have no idea.

Christina started to cry, and I paused for a few moments and then continued the meditation. "You will come into both the sperm and the egg, but your spirit enters one just a little before it enters the other. Just notice which one you come into first." I then took her step by step through the path of first the egg and then the sperm, leading up to their moment of meeting.

"Now I want you to feel the nucleus of the sperm cell be-

Hands
of
Life

ing pushed closer and closer to the nucleus of the egg by the egg's protoplasm," I told Christina. "When they fuse, any damage done to the sperm's DNA in the long journey to the egg will be repaired. About twenty-four hours after the moment of conception, the first great division of one cell into two will occur." As I said this, I put my hand on the center of her chest. "Just observe how you feel about this splitting. And then feel two cells splitting into four, and four into eight, and eight into sixteen, as you start rolling down the fallopian tube toward the great space of the uterus." It was this tumbling, this journey toward implantation, that I had seen when I was working in Angelica's surgery as the surgeon was putting in the new saline implant.

"At the end of the fallopian tube there is a sphincter. The cells surrounding and supporting the fertilized egg and its sister cells now secrete progesterone, which causes the sphincter to open just enough for you to squeeze through. This is, in fact, your first experience of what birth will be like.

"Now that you are in the great space of the uterus itself, you must find a place to implant so you can be nurtured. Notice how welcoming or how rejecting the wall of the uterus feels to you. Is it like plush red velvet inviting you to sink in? Or is it hard, rough, and unwelcoming? In either case you have only seven days in which to implant, or you will die. Do you stay in one place, or do you have to move to find another that is more accommodating?" When I did this exercise, I found that I had to move a couple of times along the wall of my mother's uterus before I could find a place where I could really sink in. It later occurred to me that my habit of changing tables at a restaurant and frequently feeling that wherever I am seated is not quite the right place for my comfort might be related to this.

"Now feel yourself burrowing into the uterine wall much as the sperm burrowed into the egg. Feel yourself breaking through the walls of your mother's capillaries to reach the rich arterial blood spiraling down to you. And feel the wall of the uterus closing over you, sealing you inside. You are completely part of her. You know everything about her, even though she doesn't even know you're there. Every breath she takes is your breath, and every beat of her heat is your heartbeat.

"Feel yourself inside the uterine wall, and feel if you are being nourished as you need to be," I said to Christina. "And now feel yourself growing, pushing back out through the wall into the vast space of the uterus itself, attached only by a tiny stalk that will become the umbilical cord." At this point she curled up into a fetal position and began to shake. "What's happening? I asked.

"It's very dark, and it's very cold," she said. "I'm very frightened."

I wanted to take her all the way through to her birth, but we were running out of time, and I still needed to take her through the surgery. I ended the meditation therefore at the end of the first trimester, with the nerve cells and muscle cells meeting and her first directed movement inside her mother's body. We both felt that her mother experienced this quickening with distaste and alarm.

I told Christina that we could continue this work during the surgery. She might very well go back to other memories inside the womb and I would be there to help her process them. She was very excited about this possibility and about the potential for healing that the whole event presented. "I'm actually looking forward to it," she told me. "I never thought I'd find myself saying that!" Another energy healer who had been working with her and who wanted to work in surgery would also be there, working at her feet.

Christina's surgeon was Elizabeth Clark, and when she came to see Christina shortly before we went into the operating room, I was struck by the warmth of their connection. Dr. Clark seemed completely at ease with my presence there and very open to ideas about the body's energy—so much so that she asked me to do a little quick energy work on her very pregnant body, and I happily obliged.

In the operating room, just as Christina was going under, I whispered to her to go as far back as she needed to for her optimum healing. This turned out to be a big mistake, because to the anesthesiologist's surprise and horror, instead of becoming motionless, she began moving her pelvis back and forth in jerky movements as if thrusting something from her. She needed more anesthesia than he had anticipated from her very calm state upon entering the OR, and he started pumping it into her. "I really don't understand this!" he said.

"I think I can explain," I said, deciding to risk being taken for an utter lunatic. "Just as she was going under, I told her to go as far back in her history as she needed to for her own healing. I think she went straight back to the womb when I said that, because those movements are what people who study prenatal influences on adult life have identified as 'umbilical affect.' It's a reaction to the feeling of something toxic coming in through the umbilical cord." The anesthesiologist was quite intrigued by this explanation, and so when he tried to put the breathing tube down and her throat tightened up, I felt comfortable telling her out loud that this was another experience of trauma in the umbilical cord. Her throat relaxed immediately.

When Dr. Clark removed the lump, I told Christina that all her mother's bitterness about nurturing would leave her body with it. The lump also seemed to hold her mother's rage at her own mother. I couldn't get over the feeling that the cancerous tissue that was being removed was like fetal tissue—less differentiated than normal cells and growing very quickly—and that the surgery was a reenactment of Christina's mother's desire to be rid of what was growing inside her.

I made the mistake of mentioning this to the others in the OR, and the anesthesiologist's response was "Lots of people have difficult childhoods, but they don't get cancer." When he said this, I got a feeling that Christina's body was wracked with sobs. I leaned over and whispered in her ear that the anesthesiologist, like her father, was trivializing her pain, but that I knew how much she had suffered and I took it very seriously. I felt her despair turning to anger.

Perhaps by coincidence, but probably not, Christina took an unusually long time to come out of the anesthesia, much to the frustration of the anesthesiologist, who kept calling her name and telling her to wake up. I felt quite certain that this was her way of showing her anger at him.

In the recovery room I asked her what the surgery was like for her. "It was like I went back to some very watery place," she said.

I talked to the other healer about her experience, and she told me that she had had some trouble staying connected to Christina. I told her my perception of where Christina had traveled and her emotions along the way and suggested that this might be a place in her own life that she was not prepared to return to yet. The challenge for a healer working in surgery, I think, has very little to do with the technology of the surgery itself and very much to do with her own emotional journey.

Since this was a professional niche that I had virtually created, I was seized with a terrible sense of responsibility. How could I, even when training healers to go into surgery, guarantee that they would have the emotional sophistication to deal with everything that was happening on an emotional as well as a physical level with both the patient and the staff? How humiliating for me if healers went in to do this work who didn't know everything that I knew! What would the surgeons say if the healers gave anything less than a brilliant performance?

I calmed myself with the reflection that people would bring into surgery the healers they needed to have there and that whatever happened would increase everybody's information about the process.

Chapter Fourteen

WHERE SHOULD HEALING START?

Before coming to California, I had gotten a call from Stephanie Taylor, an obstetrician-gynecologist and obstetric surgeon from Monterey who had heard tapes of my lectures and was interested in my work. After I arrived, she graciously offered to drive up to San Francisco to meet with me, and I was immediately taken with her intelligence, her energy, her enthusiasm, and her sense of mission. She had been a neurochemist before becoming a doctor and was very much in sync with my ideas about the macro-micro relationship in which organ malfunction inside the body mirrors organelle malfunction inside the cell. A teacher of tai chi, she was also testing out whether the revolution in health care could get a foothold in Monterey.

Her plan was to bring me down to the community hospital in Monterey to address the surgical nursing staff. They were open to anything that would help the patients, she said. I said I'd be glad to come down if she could arrange for me to work on a couple of breast cancer surgeries while I was there. I'd also love to be present at a birth, if it could be arranged. She said she had no patients on the verge of delivery, but she might have a pelvic surgery scheduled during that time period, and she'd be glad to have me attend and work with the patient.

The Monterey Peninsula has more miles of fairway than any other comparable area in the world, and rumor has it that the first doctors who came to the very beautifully sited community hospital did so in order to perfect their golf game. Stephanie, in her forties (and seeming, with her bangs and pigtail and bubbling enthusiasm, much younger) was part of a newer wave of physicians who were slowly challenging the domination of the old guard. The hospital lobby, with its huge marble goldfish pool surrounded by comfortable chairs and couches and little tables where one could eat, reminded me more of a resort hotel than a medical facility. Nor was this just an aesthetic facade. The operating rooms actually had windows through which one could see a landscape of hills dotted with evergreens. Anyone who happened to die in the one of these ORs would definitely feel he had been granted a glimpse of heaven on his way out.

I worked in two breast cancer surgeries there and was surprised that the older of the two surgeons seemed the more open to what I was doing. Stephanie, however, was not surprised. "He has a reputation for really caring about his patients," she said. "He regularly calls them at home after the surgery, and they adore him."

PELVIC ADHESIONS

As predicted, Stephanie had a pelvic surgery to perform, which she would do with the help of a laparoscope—a tube with a camera on the end that allows the surgeon to see inside the peritoneal cavity. The tube is inserted through an incision near the navel, but the significance of this didn't strike me until we were well into the surgery.

The patient, a woman in her twenties named Ellen, had been suffering from severe lower abdominal pains. The purpose of the surgery was to remove suspected adhesions between the uterus and the intestines. The anesthesiologist told her that she would "have a nice rest," but a wave of nausea came into her chest followed by terror. It subsided immediately when the anesthesiologist very gently touched the side of her face. I was struck by the power of this simple act.

I told Ellen, once she was under, "Be inside your mother," and felt panic rising in her throat. I got an image of her parents fighting during the pregnancy and her father violently attacking her mother. The gas that was injected into the peritoneal cavity brought up memories of her mother's nausea during the pregnancy, and the insertion of the laparoscope caused pelvic contractions. As Stephanie started poking the adhesions—strands of whitish connective tissue clearly visible on the video monitors—a feeling of "I don't want to be here" came up in Ellen, and I got images of the implantation journey and implantation itself, which seemed very difficult.

The adhesions, I suddenly realized, represented the desperation of her efforts to stay attached to her mother in utero and her knowledge that her very existence was causing her mother pain. As a way of reenacting this situation, she had created in her own body something clinging to her uterus that was causing her pain. A tremendous feeling of relief swept through her when the adhesions were cut, and I knew that it was not just the physical act of cutting but the flow of loving feeling from Stephanie's hands that was doing the healing.

Several weeks later I was relaxing in the sun on a bench outside Stanford University Hospital in Palo Alto, having just finished working on a mastectomy there, when a familiar figure strode by. It was Denise Mark, a well-known holistic physician from San Francisco, nicknamed "the Natural Hormone Queen" because she guides perimenopausal and menopausal women to natural alternatives to the standard hormone replacement therapies.

I had already met Denise, shortly after coming to San Francisco. Over dinner she had described to me her conversion from the rigidities of orthodox medicine to a broader path and the parallels between her spiritual journey and her professional life. She had been working with Camran Nezhat, she said, the Stanford surgeon who had invented video laparoscopy and was the world's leading expert in the field. She thought he might be open to the idea of a healer in the operating room and had suggested the two of us get together sometime.

ENDOMETRIOSIS

Dr. Nezhat, an extremely handsome and charming man, was walking with her that day in Palo Alto. As I walked with them back to his office, we both remarked on the coincidence of this chance meeting. His specialty is endometreosis, a condition in which pieces of the uterine lining (or endometrium) detach themselves and adhere to the outside of the uterus, the ovaries, and sometimes the intestines. In surgery they are burned off with a laser, and in some cases the endometrium itself is partly lasered away. For reasons that no one has been able to explain, there is a twenty percent recurrence rate.

I told him about the surgery I'd worked on in Monterey and my idea that the patient was recreating inside her body a model of her own experience in the womb. "I have a hunch that endometriosis is related to prenatal life as well," I said.

"It would be interesting to interview women with the condition and see if those in whom it recurs had a higher level of prenatal trauma," he said.

"Yes. The problem is that, except through regression, they

Hands
of
Life

2 7 1

won't remember. And their mothers may not be willing to be candid with them about their feelings during the pregnancy. Still, it would also be interesting to see if a healer working on, say, a hundred cases with you and helping the women to process what came up for them emotionally during the surgery could substantially reduce the recurrence rate."

Denise mentioned that she had a patient coming in for surgery with Dr. Nezhat in the next couple of weeks. The surgery was for endometriosis and would involve burning off some of the unusually thick lining of the uterus, which it was believed might be causing the problem. Dr. Nezhat would be removing the appendix, which showed signs of inflammation, as well. Denise suggested that I work with the patient so that he and I could get a sense of what it would be like to work together.

April, Denise's patient, was a pale, blond, overweight woman in her early forties; her troubled complexion indicated to me a need to discharge toxins from her body. The dark circles under her eyes showed a depletion of kidney energy, which in terms of Chinese medicine would be consistent with problems in any area of the body involved with sexuality. What did she know about her own gestation and birth? I asked. "The birth was induced," she said. "And I know that my mother had an epidural," which meant that she was cut off from most sensation in her lower body during the birth. I put my hands over April's first and second chakras, the centers of survival and sexuality and creativity, and felt a dense rage in the energy field.

The severe pain she had with her menstrual periods, she told me, began when she was twenty. "My parents were getting a divorce, and there was a lot of turmoil."

In the operating room I put my thumbs on the points that stimulate kidney energy on the soles of her feet. Although in Chinese medicine the kidneys are believed to normally hold fear, at a deeper level they also hold profound grief, and this was what I felt coming back at me. Once April was under, I put my hand over her lower abdomen again and noticed that the energy in the second chakra had moved from anger to love.

Before the surgery actually began, my eyes swept over the very impressive-looking video setup that Dr. Nezhat was busy explaining to a group of visiting physicians from a variety of countries. His delight in the brilliance of the technology was evident, but once his explanation was over, it did not keep him from focusing with genuine warmth and interest on the patient herself. He talked to her soothingly and kept up the discourse, which was recorded, along with the surgery, throughout the whole procedure.

My mind, however, had gone down a different track. I looked at all the equipment and thought of the equipment in all the other operating rooms I had been in: the cameras, the video machines, the X-ray machines, the bypass machines, the ultrasound devices, the anesthesia machines, the electric cauterizers, the headlamps, the monitors, the paddles. Then my mind jumped to computer-guided missiles, radar screens, and bombers. God, we were good at creating technology, I thought again—and especially good at creating medical technology and military technology. And we were willing to spend billions of dollars on this technology just to avoid having feelings.

The proliferation and escalating costs of both medical technology and military technology actually represent the massive failure of human technology. In the case of medicine, it represents the failure to resolve conflicts within the self. In the case of military technology, it is the failure to resolve conflicts with others. What would happen, I wondered, if the vast resources being poured into medical technology were applied to support and help parents and children in their struggle to work through their pain and love each other?

Actually, I would be content if they just defunded the National Institutes of Health and put all the money into poverty programs or boosting education in poor neighborhoods. I could almost guarantee a rise in the nation's health indices. And if the military budget were largely diverted into similar programs abroad, the security of the world would be substantially enhanced.

A nurse swabbed the lower part of April's body with betadine, and an image of her as a baby being bathed came to me. I wished I understood the mechanisms of anesthesia better—I wished that anyone understood them—so that I might gain some understanding of why people travel back so quickly when they are under. Perhaps the simple fact that they are physically helpless and vulnerable triggers memories of other situations in which this is the case.

The next thing I felt was a sorrow in April's right ovary, which was probably the ovary in her mother's body from which the egg that became April was released. I concluded this because the feeling was followed by a sense of turmoil around her implantation in the wall of her mother's womb and a sense that her mother didn't want her. This feeling was probably reactivated during her parents' divorce, which was when her menstrual pain began.

When the laparoscope went in at a point near the navel, I understood how every part of the surgery is unconsciously designed to stimulate and reactivate prenatal trauma. Dr. Nezhat first worked on removing April's appendix, which was filled with terror at being forced to leave the body. When he told April what he was doing, there was sorrow and weeping and a sense of helplessness in the organ. It seemed to mirror April's own sense as a fetus of being something unnecessary and unwanted. There was momentary relief when the appendix was first completely excised, and then sorrow and regret in April's body.

Dr. Nezhat then went in through the vagina to remove a cyst inside the ovary, and a wave of sexual shame swept through April's body. Whether this was about some abuse she herself had suffered or an abusive sexual relationship between her parents was not clear to me. Perhaps it was about both. There was also a sense of the embryo struggling to survive in the womb and not getting enough nourishment. When he actually entered her vagina with the laser, there was an explosion of energy in her head and a sadness in the uterus.

When the cyst was removed, Dr. Nezhat proceeded to remove a layer of April's unusually thick endometrium. It occurred to me that she was having cut out of her own body the part of her mother that had rejected her. The reason she had created this very thick uterine lining, I thought, was to create in her body the kind of uterine wall she would have wanted as a conceptus—thick, welcoming, and filled with nurturing blood.

The anesthesiologist remarked on how gently April came out of the anesthesia, but I was troubled that she experienced a great deal of lower abdominal pain in the recovery room. I felt it was rage, but my discussion with her before the surgery alerted me that her anger at her family was not something she would be comfortable confronting. She would rather endure physical pain and further deaden the emotions by covering the area with a thick layer of fat than risk connecting with her rage at what she had experienced as a child. It felt less dangerous.

As I have said, I am confronted with this kind of situation over and over again in my work, and it is a source of continuing frustration to me. Most people who have gone to all the trouble of creating a serious physical problem in their bodies are too terrified of the alternative—the open acknowledgment and expression of their feelings—to embrace it. From a very early age, they have been humiliated over and over again by physical or verbal abuse and punished for any attempt to defend themselves against that humiliation. Moreover, the right of people in power to humiliate people who have no power is ingrained in may of our social structures.

I used to take it very personally that my love, my caring, and my insights were not enough to cause a complete turnaround in patients. I gradually began to believe that I had to attack the problem on a different level and work at creating a social climate where emotional intactness is not the aberration but the norm.

Social Healing

Before leaving New York, I had come up with a plan to teach energy healing to inner-city teenagers and then bring them into hospitals with me to work with patients under my direction. I thought that the two groups had a great deal in common, both being isolated from the normal flow of life and more or less isolated from the rest of society. And both, in their own way, expressed the violence to which they had been subjected.

"Are you crazy, Julie?" a friend of mine who works for the mayor of San Francisco had said just before I left. "Nobody reaches those kids." That was all I needed to hear.

"Do you think some middle-class white guy with a heart attack is going to want to see a bunch of black kids in Reeboks, with their caps turned around, putting their little black hands on his body in the ICU?" another friend, who had served for years on a hospital board, asked me. "He'll probably have another attack, then and there!"

Just as many people I spoke to, however, thought that it was a wonderful idea. Something pleased me about taking the big guns of the New Age and aiming them at the ghetto. The year before I had made something of a start at this.

In a neglected neighborhood of Brooklyn, a former New York City policeman had started a karate school for kids to keep them off drugs and out of gangs. One early evening I drove out along the Brooklyn-Queens Expressway and then under it, through sad and shabby streets, until I came to the address, a storefront on one of the avenues.

Inside was a large room with a little raised area for sitting at the front and dressing rooms behind. Here I found Joseph

Lopez, the director of the school—or "Joelowe" as he is lovingly known by his students and their parents.

My first impulse had been to work with the most difficult, most dangerous kids because they seemed to be the ones most desperately in need. But they also represented the highest potential for failure, and that was clearly not the way to begin. It made more sense to start with kids who already had some focus on changing their lives. Then perhaps they could help me figure out how to reach the others.

I watched about twenty teenagers go through their exercises under Joelowe's direction. His patience and dedication were obvious, and even the kids who were having trouble being completely present, who didn't do the exercises well, and who wore sullen or resentful expressions on their faces for much of the time, slowly soaked up this caring feeling from him and at the end of the two hours were a little more comfortable in their bodies.

When the class was over, Joelowe introduced me to the students and to the parents who had gathered to watch them or to pick them up. I talked about my work and how it related to karate. "The energy that Joelowe is disciplining you to use to defend yourselves is the same energy I use in healing. I'd like to teach you how to use it in that way as well." I went on to explain about the chakras and the acupuncture meridians as places in the body where energy is concentrated and through which it is transported.

"So if you hurt your knee in an exercise, you might want to have someone touch places on your liver meridian. You also might want to remember what you were thinking about just before you hurt your knee, because thoughts and feelings carry energy as well."

They were raptly attentive and, when I finished talking, full of questions. Before I left, one of the mothers came up to me and asked if I could help her with her headaches, which she believed were caused by tension. "Perhaps I could teach your son how to heal your headaches. Children are always trying to heal their parents, but sometimes parents don't see this." Clearly one of my challenges would be to get parents to value their children's energy, rather than fighting it or trying to control it. But by having the children work on their parents and friends as part of their "homework," I saw, the school could become a vortex of healing for the whole neighborhood.

I promised Joelowe that when I had raised the money to put a healing program in place, I would come back. I planned to focus on experimental work with teenagers in this and other settings when my work in San Francisco was finished. A month before I left San Francisco, a patient told me about a friend of hers who was also working with disadvantaged kids in an innovative way. I decided to make that program the focus of my work for the summer.

When I got back to New York, I got in touch with Peter Rose, who runs Clearpool, an organization that has set up alternative schools in three inner-city New York neighborhoods and also maintains a rural campus for the children in Carmel, about an hour north of the city, close to where I live. I visited Peter at the Carmel site, which was formerly a summer camp, now filled to the brim with children, mostly African-American and Hispanic, from Bedford Stuyvesant in Brooklyn and from the South Bronx.

I was enchanted with the feeling of the place and with Peter, his wife Jocelyn, and Christa Towne, who was in charge of Clearpool's rural facility. My patient from San Francisco who had told me about Clearpool gave Peter a healing session with me as a present. When I worked on him, focusing on the tension in his back, I saw that the compassion he extended so tirelessly to the children at Clearpool needed to be given to himself and to the oppressed child within him.

Since my interest was in teenagers, we agreed that I would do some workshops with the teenage interns working at Clearpool. Before I left the administration building where I had been meeting with Peter, I saw two young boys sitting silently in chairs, their eyes cast down. "They were fighting," Peter told me. "I'm going to talk to them."

Driving home, I was overwhelmed with the enormity of Peter's task: to change the way poor children are educated. Surgery was simple by comparison, I thought. Perhaps I was crazy to want to join in any way in this effort. What made me think I could really have an impact? Why not just keep doing what I was doing? Wasn't trying to change the way surgery is done in this country enough?

But I was back the following week, teaching thirty inner-city teenagers how to sense the energy around the body, how to test the strength of chakras, and, by example, how to translate some of those energetic messages into emotional truths. I found it thrilling. After some initial shyness and joking around, they become truly engaged in the process, and every one of us could feel the energy in the room getting stronger as we kept working together. I was also excited by the depth of their feeling for each other, which I was certain had been nurtured by being at Clearpool together and having responsibility for younger kids. Finally, they exhibited a great deal of skill at tuning in to each other during the one-on-one exercises, and they themselves were excited about what they could pick up and transmit. *It's going to work,* I thought. *It's really going to work.*

As an opening exercise, I had them look around the circle in which we were sitting and choose someone they really liked or were attracted to at that moment. "Don't worry," I said. "You're not going to have to tell us who it is. Now I want you to close your eyes and just feel that person's energy—whatever that means to you." I gave them a couple of minutes. "Now open your eyes, look around again, and find someone you don't like or don't trust—just at this moment. Now close your eyes, and take a few moments to feel that person's energy.

"What was that like for you?" I asked a chubby girl of about fourteen dressed in overalls, sitting next to me.

"When I felt the energy of the person I liked, I sort of relaxed all over my body," she said. "With the person I didn't like, I felt something like a wall that I couldn't get through." Then I asked each of them in turn to share. A couple of them mentioned that the energy of the person they didn't like felt exactly like their own. I congratulated them on being so adept at sensing energy, and then we went around the circle again, with each person sharing his or her name and one thing about themselves that they would like to change. A couple of the overweight girls mentioned their weight. One boy said that he would like to be able to concentrate better on his schoolwork and stop disappointing his mother. Another mentioned, with real terror in his voice, his fear that he would not be able to change—would not be able to stay in school, graduate, get a job, and make anything out of his life.

When the sharing was over, I asked them to close their eyes again and once more feel the energy of the person they thought they didn't like or didn't trust. "It felt real different this time," a girl sitting across the room volunteered. "Before, this person's energy felt very dark and scary. Now it felt light, not dangerous at all." Just about everyone agreed that there had been an energy shift of this kind since the sharing.

In the second session, which Peter and Jocelyn also attended, I had them do an exercise to experience how energy and information are transmitted through the eyes and through the hands. Working in pairs, I told them that they were going to communicate a secret, but without talking. The moment I said it, I could feel the fear level rise in the room. Everyone was instantly engaged. "Think of something that's really important to you and that you normally wouldn't tell anybody," I said. "And don't worry—you're not going to be asked to say out loud what it is. Now, looking into your partner's eyes, I want you to communicate that secret just with the energy of your eyes." I gave them a few minutes. Then I had them do the same exercise again, this time with their eyes closed but their hands touching palm to palm. I told them to send the energy and the information of the secret through their hands. Then I had them open their eyes and do both together. Most people agreed that the feeling was much stronger when both the hands and the eyes were engaged, but everybody felt something under each of the three conditions. They shared what they'd experienced with each other. Then they switched roles. Many of them discovered that their partner got the essence and in some cases even the details of their secret—such as whom it was about. A couple of the girls were in tears.

Before I'd started working at Clearpool, Peter had warned me that I might have some trouble getting a couple of the kids with fundamentalist Christian beliefs to go along with what I was doing. When one of them, an attractive young man of nineteen in dreadlocks, asked me where the power of the energy came from, I said that I really didn't know but that touching someone with a loving intent seemed to summon it. "And Christ promised his disciples that what he did, they also would be able to do. I think healing was one of the things to which he was referring when he said this."

Later, after the last session was over, he told me, "When you first started, I didn't trust this stuff. But then I really felt the energy—felt it myself, in my own body. Discovering this work is like having your first sexual experience. Afterward nothing is the same." It was the greatest compliment I had ever received.

BACK TO THE BRAIN

I made plans to work with some at-risk teenagers in Poughkeepsie during the fall, but my resolution to focus exclusively on this work and to stay out of operating rooms for a while was shaken when I got a phone call from Tracy, with whom I had worked in such an exciting way around her mastectomy over a year earlier. "Luke," she said, referring to her nine-year-old son, "has a pineal gland tumor. He's going in for surgery. Will you help?"

There was no way I could turn Tracy down. Luke was, in a sense, an ideal patient, both because of Tracy's experience of and commitment to alternative therapies and because of her willingness to entertain the idea that her relationship with her husband and her conflicted feelings about the pregnancy might be a key factor in her child's illness. Luke was also incredibly sensitive to what was going on inside his own body and had vivid images both of the tumor and of energy moving inside him.

Things moved very quickly, and I wasn't able to see Luke until the morning of the surgery. Beforehand I researched embryology and the development of the brain to see what I could learn about the pineal gland. I discovered that it is formed in the seventh week after conception. I asked Tracy what was going on in her life at the time.

"I had just missed my second period. When I missed the first one, because I didn't want to be pregnant, I thought, 'This really doesn't mean anything.' When I missed the second one, there was no longer any doubt. I thought, 'Oh shit, I'm not ready for this.' I was also afraid, for some reason, that this pregnancy would make my husband leave me. Of course it didn't. We both adored Luke from the moment he was born. But the beginning was very difficult."

I suggested to Tracy very strongly that she tell Luke, difficult as I knew it would be for her. "Unconsciously he knows it already. When you tell him, he will feel less crazy and isolated with the information."

Upstairs in the hospital I had enough time before Luke was called down for surgery to take him through the whole procedure, which he went through very trustingly and easily. Tracy complained to me about her husband's lack of involvement— the same thing she felt had happened around her mastectomy. What I saw, by contrast, was his complete love and devotion to this child. "Tracy, you're not taking in the loving feeling he's pouring into Luke," I said. I could feel her giving up a little. I also observed her sense of isolation—her feeling that she had to do everything herself, like single-handedly manage Luke's care and insure his recovery. It was difficult to tell how much of this feeling was based on an unalterable reality of her marriage and how much of it she was creating. In either case I ached for her. I also realized that this sense of isolation was something Luke shared.

Waiting in the crowded corridor outside the operating room, I put my hands on Luke's head and felt tremendous rage in his brain. It was like the feeling I had had working with Walter—the sense that the brain was trying to do the body's work by holding anger for it instead of allowing the body to take that anger into action. There was also a feeling of sorrow and isolation.

Inside the OR, remembering my experience with Christina, I waited until Luke was completely sedated before telling him, "Go back as far as you need to go for healing." Immediately I felt rage come up and almost a scream of "Let me out of here!" This was followed by a great sorrow in his chest, which I identified as Tracy's despair during the pregnancy. I told him to release all of Tracy's sorrow from his body, and he immediately felt lighter. "We're going to find out what happened in your first seven weeks inside your mother," I said, and terror ran through him. This was followed by a feeling of "I'm going to make it, no matter what," which came up as they were shaving and prepping his head, and a bolt of rage as the pins went in to hold it still and steady during the surgery.

A sadness swirled around in the place where his womb would be if he were a girl, which I again identified as Tracy's feeling. The moment I acknowledged it, it changed to a sense of determination. I was working at Luke's feet, sometimes massaging them, sometimes just holding them, and sometimes touching various acupuncture points. The energy in the gallbladder meridian, which I felt through points in the outer edge of the nail on the fourth toe, was very strong. Because this meridian balances the liver's energy of action with an energy of knowing, it is one which I associate with the workings of the brain.

When the scope was in place, allowing the surgeons to actually see the tumor, I felt terror in the malignant tissue at being discovered and potentially killed. Did this feeling mirror Luke's own feeling in the womb at the seventh week? Tracy must have had at least some fleeting thoughts of abortion. Was the urgent growth, which cancerous tissue represented in this case, about some feeling of wanting to escape, to find a way out of an uncomfortable womb?

When a piece of the tumor was snipped off to be biopsied, energy exploded both in the tumor and in the gallbladder meridian. Every time one of the surgeons touched the tumor with an instrument, a feeling of wildly chaotic energy rippled through Luke's body. When a piece of the tumor was literally blown out by internal pressure, a tremendous sense of relief came over Luke. How desperately did this very well-behaved and quiet child want to explode? I wondered. What consequences did he fear for himself and his mother if he did so? Tracy had lived under conditions of extreme constraint as a child; how much of her frustration, for all her love of him, did she unconsciously impose upon Luke?

I asked one of the surgeons about the nature of the tumor, and he said that there was a high probability that it was a germinoma, which in its structure is like the tissue of the placenta. This made a great deal of sense to me, since the placenta is the place where mother and unborn child meet. I shared with him my idea that the tumor was related to emotional trauma during the pregnancy; because of the intake of stress hormones from the mother, I said, the trauma arrested the growth of certain cells and kept them in an undifferentiated fetal state. He said that it would be interesting to do an epidemiological study of the mothers of children with childhood tumors and see what correlations there might be between maternal stress during gestation and tumor formation.

Ten days after the surgery, Luke and his parents came to see me for a postoperative session. Luke looked pale and tired and had been feeling weak. I also got a feeling that he had not decided yet that he really wanted to stay here. I sensed a surge of infant anger in him and asked him to lie down on the floor and kick his legs like a baby. His father was frightened that this would wear him out, but the energy started to move down his legs as he did so, and I felt confident that he would be more energized.

I then took all three of them through a prenatal regression meditation. Luke and his father relaxed into it easily, but Tracy had trouble with it because, as she later told me, she couldn't decide whether to reexperience her own gestation or Luke's.

At the end of the session, I was still left with the feeling that Luke had not decided whether he wanted to live or die, and I told them so. My private conclusion was that he felt, despairingly, that he might have to go so far as to leave his parents to demonstrate to them the damage that the dislocation and hypocrisy in their relationship and the desperation in their individual lives was inflicting on him. He might have to go that far to heal them.

In preparation for chemotherapy, I suggested to Luke that he spend the time when the chemicals were coming into his body consciously traveling back to life inside his mother's body when she was pregnant with him. "She was under a lot of pressure," I told him. "The chemo will stress your system the way the stress hormones from her body did at that time. This will be a chance for you to release the memory of that stress from your body."

Tracy told me later that when they got home, even her husband, who had been skeptical about my work, admitted that Luke seemed to have more energy and looked much better.

Tracy, who was doing daily jin shin jitsu treatments on Luke, kept me posted about his progress. The doctors were amazed that, except for hair loss, he had virtually no side effects from the very heavy doses of chemotherapy. He regularly went inside his head to visit his tumor and did an anatomically correct drawing of it without ever having seen a picture of it.

About two months after the initial operation, he was scheduled for a relatively minor surgery to put in a mediport, which would allow them to administer chemotherapy without constantly reopening a vein. Tracy called to ask me if I could work on this surgery with him as well, and we arranged for a preoperative session at my house a few days beforehand. Her husband was busy, she said, so she and Luke would be coming on their own this time. She had not yet told Luke about her experience of the pregnancy.

Before they arrived, I had decided that the most essential thing was for Luke to work on releasing his anger, especially his anger at Tracy. I mentioned this to her on the phone, and she was completely open to it although she admitted that she was a little scared. When I saw them, however, the overwhelming feeling coming from Luke was pain, which I felt was connected to his desire to protect and take care of Tracy. When I mentioned this, Tracy told me how guilty she'd been feeling that Luke was the one who had been comforting and reassuring her. "He keeps telling me, 'Don't worry, Mommy. Everything's going to be all right,' " she said.

"Just look at him," I said, "and take in his feeling."

She did, and began to cry. "I feel I should be taking care of him, not the other way around," she protested.

"If you take care of yourself, then Luke won't have to take care of you. But you can't control his impulse to care for you. Would you like to tell Luke how you felt when you knew that you were pregnant with him?"

"I was very frightened. I didn't think I was ready for it, and I was afraid I might die." I could feel relief moving through

Luke's body as she said this, and love pouring out from him to his mother.

Tracy sat on my couch with her legs up, and Luke leaned back against her. I did some energy work at his feet and then took him through the surgery. I told him again that the chemotherapy would allow him to experience what his mother was feeling and what she was sending into his body during the pregnancy, and that he could use it to heal them both from the trauma of that experience.

As they were driving home in the car, Tracy, hardly an unbiased observer, wanted to know what Luke experienced during the session and how he felt afterward. "I usually feel a very light, floating feeling after I work with her," she prompted.

"Yes, I feel light," he said, "and very relaxed. I also felt a fist inside my head open and release some of the anger."

Tracy had gotten permission to go into the operating room with Luke and stay until he was anesthetized. I felt terror in him until Tracy, following my suggestion, put her hand on the middle of his chest. At that point it melted away. The terror rose again as the needles for the IV lines went in. This time it felt like sexual terror, and I had a flash of Tracy's fear of sexual penetration.

The anesthesiologist seemed to me to be handling Luke rather roughly. Instead of going into my usual state of inner seething, I found myself saying out loud to Luke, "Everyone in here who touches you, touches you with love as well as wisdom. And everything that touches and enters your body touches and enters to heal. I want you to feel that love for you and feel all they know about healing you, which is also their love coming into your body."

Once Luke was under, I got an image of an infant in a crib fussing. He was being ignored and was very angry about it. I told him to move the anger down his body and feel it as power. He experienced the burning of the Bovie as a sensual feeling, and his heart reacted to the feeling of the wire going into the vein as if it were being gently and lovingly tickled. I watched everything the surgeon was doing, including the very routine stitching at the end of the surgery, with the utmost focus and fascination.

When I thought about this later, I realized that by affirming to the surgical staff as well as to Luke that they were touching him with love, I made it possible for them to openly risk that feeling in their work, which in turn made it easier for me to focus on what they were doing. The anesthesiologist commented that Luke came in very calm and that he was able to go very light on the anesthesia. I thought about his own light and smiled.

Weeks later Tracy told me that not only had Luke continued to avoid the more devastating effects of the chemo, but that all traces of the tumor had disappeared after the second round of treatments instead of after the fourth, which was the more usual case. She also told me that she had started to openly confront the issues in her marriage and was determined to resolve them.

Back to the Streets

A few months later, I finally returned to Brooklyn to fulfill my promise to Joelowe. The karate class had grown and now included about thirty young people, ranging in ages from ten to twenty-two. I told them I would be doing a six-week pilot program and started out with some of the same exercises I had done with the Clearpool interns.

Two things about this group jumped out at me. One was how difficult it was for them to maintain eye contact. The first time I asked them to look into someone else's eyes, most of them kept breaking out into nervous laughter and had to look away. The kind of focused fear you need to steadily take in a feeling from another person's eyes was very difficult for them to tolerate.

The second thing that surprised me—but that later made total sense—was how difficult it was for them to get to a connected anger feeling. When we went around the room and I asked them to share something about themselves that they didn't like or wanted to change, a number of them mentioned an impulse to violence whenever they were upset. "Someone says something mean to me, and I want to hit him," one kid said. A number of others agreed. But when I asked for a volunteer to do an anger exercise, none of the three muscular young men who tried could get the words "I'm angry" out of their mouths. "It's too embarrassing," one of them said. These were guys who had been throwing people to the floor just half an hour before.

Violence was easy, but owning their anger was difficult. In fact, it was probably because their parents instilled in them the sense that they were not entitled to their anger that they discharged it in violent and ultimately self-destructive ways.

Similarly they lived with fear, but to stay present with that feeling and take in information about whether another person was safe or dangerous was forbidden. This came from years of having to deny the truths around safety and danger in their own families.

In our society, these issues are not limited to poor and minority populations. But if I could model a solution with these kids and their families, I could apply it anywhere. It pleased me to think that the transformation of people who were largely ignored by the majority culture could become the fulcrum for turning that culture around and healing it.

Chapter Fifteen

THE BREATH OF
THE SOUL

The grant I had expected to take me back to San Francisco did not come through because the funders were not happy about my ideas connecting prenatal life and breast cancer. Nor did they heartily embrace the fact that my work with energy led so directly to working with patients' emotions. At one of the hospitals where I worked, some surgeons had voiced their ire at my suggesting to their cancer patients that their emotional lives had something to do with their disease.

The relationship of someone like myself with most institutions will probably always be limited. Sooner or later people find out my real agenda: to bring the world of feelings into the healing process and thereby to enable people to reinhabit their own bodies as places of pleasure and love instead of pain and dread. To embrace this idea, the people running and working for those institutions would have to reevaluate the role of emotions in their own work and lives, and this notion is still far from popular.

My journey into healing has really been a journey into my body. Like so many of my patients, I abandoned my body because of what had happened to it as a child. But it was waiting for my return, and each new level of energy and emotion that I was willing to experience brought me more completely into it. Throughout my career as an energy healer, this personal experience of healing has informed everything I have done.

When I started out in the surgical phase of my work, I had only the vaguest idea that the energy in an operating room might have an effect on the patient undergoing surgery and on surgical outcomes. But it does, and this energy is the collective emotional state of everybody involved, along with all the electromagnetic output of the machines and the emotions left over from previous surgeries done in the room. Since it is impossible to "clear" the room energetically between surgeries, I have told my patients to absorb into their bodies all the healing energies in the room from all the surgeries that have previously been done there, hoping that this emphasis on the positive will neutralize everything else.

"Remember that these people work for you," I say. "Beyond that, you give meaning to their lives. Without you they would have no reason to gather here today and do the highest work of all—the work of healing. You are at the very center of this drama. The love and trust you bring with you into this room makes it safe for them to love you, and it heals them as they do so."

When the body is treated as if it were only its parts, it reacts to the surgical invasion with terror in those parts that are most directly threatened by the surgery. When I first mentioned this to physicians, I was accused of "anthropomorphizing" the body. Finally a cell biologist assured me that all the functions of the body—including sensation, emotion, and memory—exist in the individual cells.

During surgery, on a whole-body level, the patient reexperiences traumatic events from the past, triggered when a certain part of the body is touched by an instrument or the surgeon's hands, or when a chemical goes into the bloodstream. Because of the nature of surgery and anesthesia, these traumas often go back to prenatal life. Perhaps on an unconscious level people come into surgery and even select certain surgeries because of a compulsion to reactivate painful memories and try to heal them. Might this be the case with all invasive medical procedures, including powerful drugs? If so, profound healing is possible in medical situations—way beyond what is currently being done.

As time has gone on, more and more surgical nurses, anesthesiologists, and surgeons have expressed an interest in learning to do what I do. This, I hope, will be the wave of the future. Everyone who goes into medicine does so with the intent to heal the whole person and, unwittingly, to heal the broken parts of himself. Since nurturing is still considered "women's work," and therefore given low esteem in our society, this impulse is ignored or suppressed in medical education. When we begin to understand that neither mental function nor physical function is separable from emotional function, this will change.

When I hear about plans for "health care reform," something inside me groans. What is really being discussed are ways to make being sick more affordable, not really to make people more healthy. But so long as we have violent parenting and a violent society, we will have violent, expensive, and reactive medicine. They complement each other and our current style of combating violence with yet more violence.

If physicians were trained to go inside their own bodies and examine their patients empathically as well as objectively, they would get a great deal more information on both a physical and psychological level. Moreover, it is unscientific to ignore the psychological information about a patient when it is so clear that, through the workings of the hypothalamus, thought and feeling are directly translated into physical chemistry, which affects the whole body through the endocrine system, the nervous system, and the immune system. An energetic transference takes place as well, but even if it did not, the evidence for a purely chemical transference is strong enough to merit serious attention to the emotional life of every patient who enters a physician's office.

Physicians can be trained to do this, just as anyone else (such as the patients and the inner-city teenagers with whom I have worked) can, and just as anyone can master the complex tasks of reading, writing, and driving an automobile.

Wherever I have worked, people have come to realize, sooner or later, that I want to be engaged with them on the level of their feelings. This is, inevitably, where the involvement with the energy of the body leads me, and this, I believe, is the most threatening part of my work. In the 1960s the vocabulary of emotion emerged from the psychiatrist's office and came into common discourse. It has been ringing in our ears ever since, threatening, along with the liberation of women, traditionally keepers of feelings, to overthrow the social order. We are in danger of being cast into a true democracy because when we feel for ourselves, we think for ourselves. When you own your body, you own your mind.

If emotional intactness were a requirement for medical school graduation, doctors would be capable of intellectual discovery at ten times the current rate. The level of connection to their patients and their emotional satisfaction from that connection—to say nothing of their improved skills at diagnosis and treatment—would alter their entire economic relationship to their profession. In short, they would find another way, besides money, of keeping score.

With the grassroots growth of interest in and use of alternative healing modalities, the great medical revolution may well come outside of medicine completely. People could and should be healing themselves and each other. Healing should be a non-profession, and healers like myself represent a transitional phase in human development. My goal with every patient is to teach myself out of a job, and although this hasn't happened yet, I believe it is inevitable.

Our ability to heal ourselves and each other with thought, feeling, and touch may simply be part of the human gene pool—it may well be part of what enabled our ancestors to live long enough to reproduce and get us here. What is certain is that the ability to know empathically what another is feeling both physically and emotionally is essential for the success of mammals on the planet, since we have such a long period of caring for the young after birth. Mammal parents simply have to be able, without language, to intuit what their infant needs. So if you are a human and if you are a mammal alive on earth today, the chances are that you can both perceive what your fellow mammals/humans are feeling and, guided by that perception, help heal them.

Right now, unfortunately, it is still difficult for most people to make associations even between what they eat and how their body functions. We used to have a similar dissociation between what we put into the earth, the air, and the water, and what came back at us. But in the last three decades this situation has changed profoundly. The same thing will happen with our bodies. In fact, there is an intimate connection between nurturing the planet and nurturing ourselves.

Similarly, the idea that what you do and don't feel can affect your health is something most people have not taken the trouble to observe. It's just not a cultural norm yet. But as we discover that throwing money at problems works even less for chronic disease than it does for chronic poverty, more and more people will be pushed to become the experts on their own bodies. In this greater intimacy with our physical beings, we will discover the engines of our emotions, the breath of our soul.

Most chronic disease begins in the womb, and the relationship of parents to themselves, to each other, to their own parents, and to their unborn child sets the stage for that child's future health. From the point of view of disease causality, embryology is a vast unexplored area in medicine. The emotional factors in embryology are almost totally ignored, yet they are key factors in weakening the body and setting the stage for disease. I predict that prenatal life will prove particularly rich as a place to investigate origins of addiction and depression.

Our current fascination with genetics suggests that we do know that something important happens to us before birth, but our focus is misplaced. It will take tremendous individual courage on all our parts to be willing to go back and accurately experience our origins. Still, we are getting closer and closer to having that courage.

The underlying theme of all my work is uncovering the roots of violence in our lives. We will stop inflicting violence on ourselves and on others only when we are willing to go back and experience how we were hurt and humiliated, our rage at what happened, and our terror of expressing that rage. I have no doubt that these patterns begin in the womb and are reinforced in our childhood, until we become their reinforcers for ourselves.

From this point of view, our technological failure to deal adequately with chronic disease on every level of society may be a great gift. In our desire to end this violence to our bodies, we may at last extend to each other the love that gives us the courage to feel and to know ourselves completely. This is what it means to put ourselves in the hands of life.

SELECTED BIBLIOGRAPHY

Becker, Robert. *Cross Currents.* Los Angeles: Tarcher, 1990.

Becker, Robert, and Gary Selden. *The Body Electric.* New York: William Morrow, 1985.

Brennan, Barbara. *Hands of Light: A Guide to Healing Through the Human Energy Field.* New York: Bantam, 1993.

Bruyere, Roslyn L. *Wheels of Light: A Study of the Chakras.* New York: Simon & Schuster, 1994.

Burmeister, Alice, with Tom Monte. *The Touch of Healing: Energizing Body, Mind, and Spirit with the Art of Jin Shin Jyutsu.* New York: Bantam, 1997.

Calder, Nigel. *The Key to the Universe: A Report on the New Physics.* New York: Viking, 1973.

Capra, Fritjof. *The Tao of Physics: An Exploration of the Parallels Between Modern Science and Eastern Mysticism.* Boston: Shambhala, 1991.

Chia, Mantak. *Awaken Healing Energy Through the Tao.* Santa Fe, NM: Aurora Press, 1983.

Chopra, Deepak. *Quantum Healing: Exploring the Frontiers of Mind Body Medicine.* New York: Bantam, 1990.

Cohen, Bonnie Bainbridge. *Sensing, Feeling and Action.* Berkeley, CA: North Atlantic Books, 1994.

Colbin, Annemarie. *Food and Healing.* New York: Ballantine Books, 1986.

Ellis, Andrew, Nigel Wiseman, and Ken Boss. *Fundamentals of Chinese Acupuncture.* Brookline, MA: Paradigm, 1988.

England, Marjorie A. *Life Before Birth.* London: Mosby Wolfe, 1996.

Fisher, Stanley. *Discovering the Power of Self-Hypnosis.* New York: HarperCollins, 1991.

Ford, Clyde W. *Where Healing Waters Meet.* Tarrytown, NY: Station Hill Press, 1992.

Gerber, Richard. *Vibrational Medicine.* Santa Fe, NM: Bear and Co., 1988.

Gilligan, James. *Violence: Reflections on a National Epidemic.* New York: Vintage, 1997.

Gilligan, Sonja Carla. *The Heterosexuals Are Coming.* New York: Fusion Groups, 1971.

Hartley, Linda. *Wisdom of the Moving Body.* Berkeley, CA: North Atlantic Books, 1995.

Hunt, Valerie V. *Infinite Mind: Science of Human Vibrations of Consciousness.* Malibu, CA: Malibu Publishing, 1996.

Jahn, Robert G., and Brenda J. Dunne. *Margins of Reality: The Role of Consciousness in the Physical World.* San Diego, CA: Harcourt Brace Jovanovich, 1987.

Kaptchuk, Ted J. *The Web That Has No Weaver: Understanding Chinese Medicine.* New York: Congdon and Weed, 1983.

Larsen, William J. *Human Embryology.* New York: Churchill Livingstone, 1993.

Love, Susan M. *Dr. Susan Love's Breast Book*. Reading, MA: Addison Wesley, 1990.

Maciocia, Giovanni. *The Foundations of Chinese Medicine*. New York: Churchill Livingstone, 1989.

Mann, Felix. *Acupuncture: The Ancient Chinese Art of Healing and How It Works Scientifically*. New York: Random House, 1973.

Myss, Caroline. *Anatomy of the Spirit: The Seven Stages of Power and Healing*. New York: Harmony Books, 1996.

Nilsson, Lennart. *A Child Is Born*. New York: Dell Publishing, 1990.

Noble, Elizabeth. *Primal Connections*. New York: Simon & Schuster, 1993.

Northrup, Christiane. *Women's Bodies, Women's Wisdom: Creating Physical and Emotional Health and Healing*. New York: Bantam, 1994.

Rossi, Ernest Lawrence. *The Psychobiology of Mind-Body Healing*. New York: W. W. Norton and Co., 1993.

Sharamon, Shalilia, and Bodo J. Baginski. *The Chakra-Handbook*. Wilmot, WI: Lotus Light Shangri-La, 1991.

Smith, Fritz Frederick. *Inner Bridges: A Guide to Energy Movement and Body Structure*. Atlanta, GA: Humanics New Age, 1996.

Starr, Paul. *The Social Transformation of American Medicine*. New York: Basic Books, 1982.

Talbot, Michael. *The Holographic Universe*. New York: HarperPerennial Library, 1992.

Tomatis, Alfred A. *The Conscious Ear*. Tarrytown, NY: Station Hill Press, 1991.

Upledger, John E. *A Brain Is Born.* Berkeley, CA: North Atlantic Books, 1996.

Vollmar, Klausbernd. *Journey Through the Chakras.* Bath, U.K.: Gateway Books, 1987.

Young, Arthur M. *Mathematics, Physics and Reality.* Portland, OR: Robert Briggs Associates, 1990.

Zukav, Gary. *The Dancing Wu Li Masters: An Overview of the New Physics.* New York: William Morrow and Co., 1979.

INDEX

Index

Index

Index

Index

ABOUT THE AUTHOR

JULIE MOTZ is an energy healer who has
worked in surgery at Columbia Presbyterian Medical Center in New York,
Stanford University Hospital in California, and many other hospitals across the
country. She has also lectured at Stanford and Dartmouth medical schools.
In addition to her hands-on healing
work, she has started a program, Health's
Angels, that teaches energy healing to
inner-city teenagers. She lives in Putnam
County, New York, and the San Francisco Bay Area.